LISTEN UP!

A Physician's Guide to Effectively Treating Your Hearing Loss

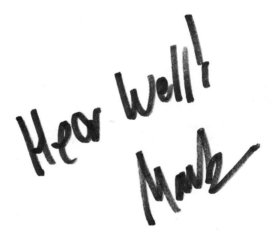

Mark J. Syms, MD

The Hearing Loss Physician

REGISTER THIS BOOK

As a thank you for buying this book I would like to give you some free gifts. This book is INTERACTIVE.

Simply visit
www.ListenUpHearing.com/register
to obtain:

- Free Video Training
- Resources and Checklists
- Free Updates to the Book

Need Help With Hearing Loss?

Schedule a Consultation With Our Team by Visiting **www.azhear.com/schedule** or call **(602) 277-HEAR (4327)**

FEEDBACK AND GUARANTEE

There may be some spelling, grammatical and layout errors. If you find one, please tell me what you find by sending me an email at m.syms@azhear.com. Just note the page number, sentence and mistake and I will fix it right away and *thank you for your help*.

If you enjoy the book, please post a review on Amazon. If you DON'T like it, send me an email, tell me why and I'll give you your money back. My direct email is m.syms@azhear.com.

Warm Regards,
Mark J. Syms, MD
The Hearing Loss Physician

For my children Matthew, Meredith, Marinna, my parents, and my patients! They all share of themselves to make me a better doctor and an even better man.

For Maria:
O, she doth teach the torches to burn bright!
It seems she hangs upon the cheek of night
Like a rich jewel in an Ethiop's ear;
Beauty too rich for use, for Earth too dear!
~William Shakespeare

"Blindness separates us from things, but deafness separates us from people."
~ *Helen Keller*

Dear Friend,

Thank you for taking the time to learn more about hearing loss. You are one step closer to effectively treating your hearing loss and improving your quality of life!

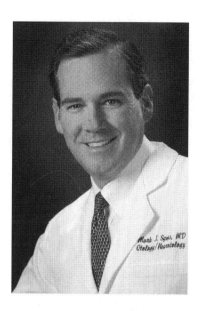

As a hearing loss physician with more than thirty years experience treating thousands of patients, I know firsthand that better hearing means a better life. I also know how time consuming, frustrating, and overwhelming it can be to find the right way to treat your hearing loss. Many patients lose hope after seeking treatment only to find their hearing is no better off and in some instances, worse.

In this book, I show you the right way to go about effectively treating your hearing loss so you can end the struggle. Too often, patients get a "quick fix" that over-promises and under-delivers. More than one in four patients with hearing aids, for example, don't use them. Here, I show you why that is and how we can do better.

You will discover exactly which questions to ask your providers so you can make an informed decision about choosing the right treatment option for you. My goal is for you to solve your hearing loss once and for all so you can remain independent, enjoy socializing, and connect better with family and friends – that is the fulfilling life you deserve.

So *Listen Up!* and let's get started on your road to better hearing and a better life!

Mark J. Syms, M.D.
The Hearing Loss Physician

DID YOU KNOW?

PERCENTAGE OF PEOPLE OVER 75
WITH DISABLING HEARING LOSS

50%

PERCENTAGE OF PEOPLE 65 TO 74
WITH DISABLING HEARING LOSS

25%

NUMBER OF U.S. ADULTS WHO COULD BENEFIT
FROM USING HEARING AIDS

28.8 million

AVERAGE COST OF UNTREATED HEARING LOSS
PER PERSON OVER A LIFETIME

$1 million

AVERAGE TIME FOR A PATIENT TO SEEK TREATMENT
AFTER BEING DIAGNOSED WITH HEARING LOSS

10 years

PERCENTAGE OF PEOPLE WITH HEARING
AIDS WHO DON'T USE THEM

25%

ARIZONA
HEARING CENTER

YOUR HEARING HEALTH
checklist

Better hearing means a better life!

- [ ] I ask people to repeat themselves often.
- [ ] I can't hear someone calling me from another room.
- [ ] People complain that I turn the television up too loud.
- [ ] I have difficulty hearing people on the telephone.
- [ ] I have difficulty understanding the dialogue at movies.
- [ ] I have trouble listening to the news on my car radio.
- [ ] I have to ask people to speak slowly to me.
- [ ] I can't understand conversations in a noisy place like a restaurant.
- [ ] It seems like people mumble a lot when speaking to me.
- [ ] I skip social events because I'm afraid I won't hear people.
- [ ] I have trouble hearing consonants.
- [ ] I have trouble hearing high pitched sounds like a doorbell.
- [ ] I am hypersensitive to certain sounds (e.g., emergency sirens, construction noise, loud music)
- [ ] I get frustrated because I can't make out what people say.
- [ ] I have ringing in my ears.

ARIZONA
HEARING CENTER

If you or a loved one experience any of the above signs of hearing loss, you should contact a hearing health care provider to set up a hearing test. This is the first step on your road to better hearing and a better life filled with family, friends, and laughter.

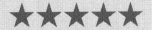

What Dr. Syms' Patients Are Saying About Better Hearing

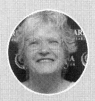

Ginger Kuberra
Payson, Arizona

"My hearing impairment caused me to be considered very shy. [People] thought I was introverted, and I'm really not! Rather than make a comment that didn't pertain to the conversation, I would keep quiet. Now with the help of Dr. Syms, I hear better and I'm all in!"

Linda Gotcher
Phoenix, Arizona

"I called my daughter crying ... I can hear! It gives you your life back. You feel like you're a part of everything. That's the one big message. If you're losing your hearing, get it checked every year. Make sure you're with someone you can trust like Dr. Syms. Don't just go to any hearing aid center. You've got to know you're with someone on the cutting edge like Dr. Syms."

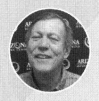

Tom Haines
Phoenix, Arizona

"Since I received my hearing aids from Dr. Syms, there's been a remarkable improvement in my ability to hear. I feel much more at ease socially and able to participate much better. It's been a remarkable breakthrough. "

Bonnie Grimm
Phoenix, Arizona

"It's a shame I waited so long to investigate [my hearing loss]. If only I had treated it years back. I was a substitute teacher at the elementary school and... [hearing loss] always held me back from improving myself. You shut yourself out even to your friends and family. You just don't feel like you're a part of anything. I thought I'd have to die like this but then we found Arizona Hearing Center and Dr. Syms and it's been remarkable to hear like I do!"

Anthony Cyplik
Phoenix, Arizona

"I suffered sudden hearing loss in my left ear and I was beginning to panic. My right ear was fine but there was no hearing at all out of my left ear. I couldn't hear anything when I put the phone up to that ear and it only created more anxiety and more panic. I knew I had to do something because all of the normal processes to clear my ear were not working. I went to see Dr. Syms and my hearing is back. I'm very thankful to Dr Syms and God above! Don't wait. The longer you wait to treat sudden hearing loss the bigger risk you have!"

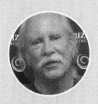

Jim Lochhead
Phoenix, Arizona

"People have been after me for years to get a hearing aid. My wife got tired of me going, 'Huh? Huh? Huh?' I couldn't hear! It was progressively getting worse and in fact, it was getting worse quicker. After seeing Dr. Syms and the folks at Arizona Hearing Center, my hearing is a lot better. I've been very happy!"

TABLE OF CONTENTS

INTRODUCTION

My Journey To Hearing Care

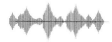

When Robby was a teenager, he was diagnosed with a brain tumor. Robby was close to his little brother, Mark. Only 8 years old at the time, Mark probably didn't understand the gravity of the diagnosis. What Mark did notice, however, was the way Robby's symptoms affected his quality of life. No tumor side effect had a greater negative impact on Robby than his hearing loss.

He wasn't only battling a life-threatening tumor. Because of his hearing loss, Robby was also unable to enjoy many things others take for granted. When Mark wanted to share a new record or go to the movies with him, it was always a challenge. The more Robby became a loner and the less he interacted with Mark, the sadder Mark became.

Doctors were able to treat the tumor, but the remaining hearing loss went untreated, which had an even worse impact on his life than the tumor itself. Mark watched as Robby struggled to play the sports he loved and interact with others. Robby suffered daily from not being able to communicate as he once did. He struggled to maintain good relationships with family and friends. Mark watched Robby transform from his outgoing big brother to an introverted, argumentative and anti-social stranger—all because of untreated hearing loss. Mark missed his fun and happy big brother.

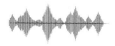

Robby's story is particularly moving and personal because I am that little brother, Mark. I lived his suffering with him and shared the frustration of his hearing loss. Robby has since passed away, and I am often reminded of the many things he missed out on. But the thing I remember most is how his hearing loss changed his personality. Robby had a good heart, but he became introverted and quick to argue; his relationships suffered. He had so much potential that was never realized—mostly because of his untreated hearing loss. As his brother, that is my most painful memory. At the time, I already knew I would become a doctor of some sort. Watching my brother's experience clarified which road I would take.

Like many following a career path, mine is based on personal experience. I saw firsthand how hearing loss affected the life of a loved one. Unlike many others, however, the person I observed was not a beloved older relative or even someone a generation above me. He was a member of my own generation, my very own sibling.

Sound As The Way To My Heart

My grandfather was a Philadelphia saxophonist, singer, and bandleader. He devoted his entire life to creating sounds that made people happy; kept them on the edge of their seats; made them sing and dance; made them feel. To him, sounds were a vehicle to deliver pleasure and emotion. The notes he conducted added up to something far greater than themselves. My grandfather sought to delight your heart through your ears. The power of sound was a lesson I learned early and deeply.

My father was a physician. He spent his days helping people become healthier. But unlike the proverbial doctor's son, my dad never pressured me into medical school. For him the title or job was not as important as being a productive member of society. But nevertheless, Dad was also blessed with a love for his job. That passion for his profession was what encouraged me to become a doctor. On occasion he got stressed out or panicked, but I never once got the impression that he regretted his career choice. Like my grandfather, Dad was lucky to find a profession that made his heart happy. He knew it. I knew it too.

How Do You Become A Good Ear Physician? Do More.

Rigorous Training

My path to becoming an ear surgeon began at Jefferson Medical College in Philadelphia. It continued with an ENT residency at Tripler Regional Medical Center in Honolulu and ear-specific fellowship training at the world-renowned House Ear Clinic in Los Angeles. After completing my training, I knew I wanted to focus on surgical procedures.

That's exactly what I did at the beginning of my career. I focused on being the best physician, technician and surgeon I could be. I never questioned the system; I tried to excel within it. Like my dad, I felt great about helping people. They came to me with a serious medical problem, and I resolved it. What could be more rewarding?

Eventually, I wanted to do more. I started to wonder if the system was *failing* patients. No single incident led me to this conclusion. It was death by a thousand paper cuts. Time and time again, I'd tell a patient during recovery, "Your surgery went very well. You need to get a pair of well-fitted hearing aids, and you'll be all set." Unless I was going to handle the hearing aid fitting myself, there was nothing more I could do. Mission accomplished, right?

Disappointing Outcomes

But far too many patients arrived at their follow-up appointment without hearing aids. It wasn't lack of diligence or willpower—they'd already made the decision to have major surgery on their ears! Clearly, they wanted to get better.

In fact, many had tried several sets of hearing aids but hadn't followed through with treatment. Common reasons were that the hearing aids didn't work or were too loud for comfort. At even the most basic level, hearing aids didn't help my patients with their hearing loss. But why not?

I decided to find out.

In-Depth Research

I had in-depth conversations with my patients. Some never even bothered with hearing aids. I asked those who'd tried hearing aids where they'd gone, what hearing aids they'd tried, and what they liked and disliked about them.

Many who purchased hearing aids complained they didn't work well enough. Often their spouse or significant other echoed that complaint. I also heard things like, "I had a friend return the hearing aids for me," "They stay in my nightstand drawer," or "My friend has hearing aids, and she says they don't work."

My patients had many misconceptions about hearing aids. Some didn't even think they had a hearing loss. Still others didn't care that they couldn't hear well. The misconceptions and miseducation were overwhelming.

A Humbling Conclusion

I realized I was part of the problem. I handed them off after surgery and thought my job was done. It was standard practice to refer these patients to an audiologist or hearing aid dispenser to discuss what came next. I assumed this process served them well. I was wrong.

These patient discussions led to a keen interest in hearing technology. I talked to physicians, audiologists, and hearing aid dispensers. I attended conferences on hearing loss and non-surgical treatment. I read audiology textbooks and the hearing loss research literature. I came to realize there had to be a better way than the current standard of treatment. Too many people showed up in my office with ineffective hearing aids.

Playing A Different Tune

My true turning point came when a friend invited me to a presentation. At the meeting, we were challenged to consider how much impact we would have over the course of our careers. As a physician, I knew I was helping people every day. But I'd never framed my own career in terms of my magnitude of impact. I started to do the math.

"I know we can do a better job serving more patients. We can develop a comprehensive, collaborative, and compassionate care model."

In my capacity as a surgeon, let's say I could operate on 500 patients each year. Over 30 years, I'd have helped 15,000 people with surgery. If I extended this beyond surgery patients, I could see around 2,000 new patients each year. This would mean I would help 60,000 patients. That's a big impact by most standards.

Remember though, many surgery patients showed up to their one-year follow-up with untreated hearing loss. How much did I really help? Is that 15,000 really 8,000? 5,000? 3,000? More importantly, could I figure out a way to help more people than I could see in 10 lifetimes? Why limit my impact to only the patients I see?

I know the hearing loss treatment system, a system of which I am a part, can do a better job serving our patients. We can develop a comprehensive, collaborative, and compassionate care model. We can keep our patients and health optimization in focus at all times. This is my goal. This is the goal of my hearing care organization, Arizona Hearing Center (www.azhear.com). This is the goal of this book.

So, Listen Up! This book will guide you and inform you, so you get the best hearing loss treatment possible. Better hearing means a better life.

CHAPTER 1

Why Most Hearing Aids Don't Work

(Hint: It's Not the Hearing Aids)

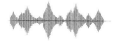

Bill was loving retirement. The lifelong workaholic was finally enjoying the benefits of all those late nights and lost weekends. He and his wife, Joanne, were in good health. They had paid off their mortgage. Their three grown children had started lives of their own. They couldn't wait to spend more time with their grandchildren. Plus, they could finally take those trips they'd been saving so long for. Life was good... Or so they thought.

There was just one tiny glitch. Bill noticed that his hearing wasn't as good as it used to be. He assumed it was from exposure to all that artillery noise during his time in the military many years ago. At first, he didn't think much of it. Then Joanne started to complain about how much he was asking her to repeat herself and look at him when talking. She'd tell him about plans to meet with friends, and he would miss the details. Joanne didn't realize he had difficulty hearing her. But then Bill became forgetful and started playing the television way too loud. After one too many missed conversations and a little coaxing from Joanne, Bill decided to get hearing aids.

They went down to their local Costco, and sure enough, Bill had hearing loss in both ears. Right away, Bill received brand new hearing aids and went on his way. Easy peasy... Or so they thought. Bill had trouble the very first week. The hearing aids were uncomfortable, sounds were too loud, and he heard a constant hum in his right ear that drove him crazy. He complained to Joanne that he didn't hear her well enough to put up with all the discomfort.

The hearing aids spent more time in their case than in Bill's ears. Needless to say, Bill became frustrated and stopped using them altogether. Bill and Joanne went about their lives as best they could, but his hearing loss made activities challenging and their retirement less enjoyable.

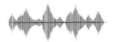

I hear this kind of story every day. Over the course of my 25-year career treating hearing loss, I have treated tens of thousands of patients with the same problem as Bill and Joanne: They shop for hearing aids the same way they shop for glasses. But hearing aids don't solve the problem, or they make it worse, or they create other problems. But why? The answer may surprise you.

Hearing loss is unique to each patient.

That's why it's my duty as a hearing care professional to focus on treating each patient's specific hearing loss. I need to consider all the medical and technological tools at my disposal. Hearing care is far more than simply dispensing hearing aids. In this and the following chapters, you'll learn why hearing aids alone don't solve the

> "It's my duty as a hearing care professional to focus on treating each patient's specific hearing loss. Hearing care is far more than simply dispensing hearing aids."

problem. You'll also start on a path to better hearing and a better quality of life. I'll discuss (1) why changing our mindset about hearing loss and its treatment is so crucial, (2) how treating hearing loss as soon as possible helps prevent dementia and ensure independence in your twilight years, and (3) how we can create a better future for those suffering from hearing loss.

Whether you're a person with hearing loss or their loved one, in these pages you'll find all the tools you need to make the right decisions about addressing hearing loss. You'll also gain insights on how to discuss hearing loss as well as information on the different treatment options. I hope you'll also find more than a few reasons to be optimistic about our potential for making hearing loss more manageable and more treated.

Treatable But Untreated

The other day, my wife was out of town visiting some friends from graduate school. They were discussing hearing loss, and someone mentioned that their hearing aids didn't work very well. My wife sent me a photo of the hearing aids and asked if I knew what the problem was. "It's not the hearing aids," I replied.

It's not uncommon for me to receive texts like these. Because I'm known as the ear guy, people want to, ahem, hear my opinion. All too often, I'm asked why somebody's hearing aids aren't doing what they're supposed to. Equally often, my answer is the same. It's not the hearing aids.

Hearing Loss is Coming for Most of Us: But it is Avoidable.

Hearing loss occupies a unique place in the history of American medicine. It's a health care issue that's been difficult to resolve for centuries, despite technological and medical advancements. Most people still suffer from hearing loss because of our broken treatment system. The established method for treating hearing loss amounts to little more than selling hearing aids. This doesn't serve patients. It also spreads bad information that should have been put to bed decades ago.

This is maddening for two reasons. First, hearing loss is pervasive. Everyone reading this book knows somebody who is affected by hearing loss. If you're over 70, there's a 50 percent chance you suffer from disabling hearing loss. In other words, we know that hearing loss is coming for more than half of us.

Second, it is entirely treatable. It's not a surprising, incurable epidemic that nobody saw coming. Yet the scourge of untreated hearing loss in older adults remains. Indeed, the age-old use of hearing loss as the punch line in a comedy routine is still commonplace.

But there is good news: We can make the impact of hearing loss minimal if we catch it early enough. Unlike other widespread diseases, such as cancer, hearing loss doesn't stump us. We usually know why it's happening and how to keep it from ruining a patient's quality of life. We have the tools, skills, and technology to treat the hearing loss of an overwhelming majority of patients.

Winning the Battle, Losing the War

We know the problem exists. We have the tools and know-how to fix it. That's half the battle – so why aren't we winning the war on hearing loss? Can you think of another condition, especially one that touches so many lives, that we basically allow to go untreated? And boy does it go untreated. According to the National Institutes of Health, only about 20 percent of people who could benefit from hearing aids wear them. That means four out of five of them drive their car, go to the movies with friends, dine at restaurants with family, talk to their grandchildren, and go to work meetings without hearing all that well. No wonder so many folks are frustrated and grouchy these days. And it's entirely fixable.

But wait, it gets worse. Of that 20 percent of people who use hearing aids, many don't receive effective treatment. Here's an example: A 2009 study from *Consumer Reports* followed 24 patients with

"We know the problem exists. We have the tools and know how to fix it. That's half the battle - so why aren't we winning the war on hearing loss?"

hearing loss as they shopped for, purchased, and used hearing aids. Each participant purchased two hearing aids during the course of the study. They wore their hearing aids in daily life for a while, then an audiologist tested their effectiveness. "Two-thirds of the 48 aids [that patients] bought were misfit: They amplified too little or too much," the report states. Imagine how frustrating that would be. You invest in hearing aids that don't work as they're supposed to, only to learn the devices weren't set up correctly in the first place.

This study only followed 24 people, but it echoes my personal experience from treating tens of thousands of people with hearing loss. If, as the study found, about one-third of people using hearing aids are getting the most from them, and if only one-fifth of people in need of hearing aids are getting them in the first place, only a pitiful 7 percent of people who might benefit from hearing aids actually benefit from them.

Again, hearing loss is not a new phenomenon. It's not one we don't know how to treat. It's one we are failing to treat.

This data raises the question I keep bringing up: Why?

Is It All About The Money?

Most people would tell you it comes down to money. It's well known that hearing aids are expensive, and most insurance doesn't cover them. In fact, only Arkansas, Connecticut, Illinois, New Hampshire, and Rhode Island require hearing aid coverage for adults. The reason for this amounts to a weird quirk of history.

In the 1960s, Medicare was being developed and enacted into law. Door-to-door salesmen sold most hearing aids. These were the same folks who sold Encyclopedia Britannica, globes, and other products. Of course, the government didn't see these people as medical professionals. When President Lyndon Johnson signed Medicare into existence on July 30, 1965, hearing aids were excluded. It's mostly remained that way ever since.

But surprisingly, in Europe, where most people can get hearing aids at no out-of-pocket cost, people still aren't using them. Only 33 percent of Europeans get their hearing loss treated. Remember, only 20 percent of people in the U.S. do. That's not a big difference. So even though cost is one reason people avoid treating their hearing loss, it's definitely not the only one.

Is It About Vanity?

Another common reason millions of Americans lose their hearing without a fight is vanity. It's even a cliché—the stubborn older adult who simply refuses to wear hearing aids. But the myths about hearing aids are outdated. They are no longer bulky, obvious devices, and the technology has outpaced popular opinion.

Plus, it's almost impossible to hide hearing loss. It sticks out just as much as the old-fashioned, clunky hearing aids. The communication struggles are obvious to family, friends, and others. They already "see" the hearing loss.

It's About The Treatment Approach

More than price or pride, the most damaging—but overlooked—factor is the very system we use to treat hearing loss. Hearing aids are often ineffective because they're seen as gadgets. The truth is they are just one part of a complete hearing health plan. Approaching hearing aids as a commodity implies they're like eyeglasses, which don't need ongoing provider support. This assembly-line mindset is the biggest obstacle to effectively treating hearing loss.

> "Approaching hearing aids as a commodity implies they're like eyeglasses, which don't need ongoing provider support. This assembly-line mindset is the biggest obstacle to effectively treating hearing loss."

In a sense, we haven't moved beyond the days of door-to-door sales. For many people, a hearing aid is one more item on their list, right after meat, trash bags, and toilet paper. Is this really the best way to treat hearing loss? Put another way, why isn't dental care available at Costco? It's because, like hearing health, dental health has a significant and life-changing impact on overall health.

Yet many people still go to a big-box retailer for hearing aids. They think they need a gadget. But a big-box store gadget won't help them communicate with loved ones *and* lower dementia risk *and* keep you out of the nursing home *and* improve overall health and quality of life. It's absurd. If I offered to perform a surgery for half price, what would you think? You would go elsewhere. Why? Because we select commodities based on price, but we select services based on quality. That's why we recoil at discounted services when our body and health are at stake.

The Wrong Way To Buy Hearing Aids

To buy a hearing aid, a prescription is required, which comes from something called an audiogram. In the traditional model, a hearing aid dispenser or doctor fills the prescription. The patient has a trial period to assess whether they like the hearing aid, and then it's theirs.

There's not a single problem in this system. There are several problems.

Many practitioners are under qualified and ill trained to fit a hearing aid correctly. It's not their fault—it's the delivery system that's built to merely provide a hearing aid, not hearing treatment and care. Dispensers, thus, offer cheaper services. Most patients don't realize they've sacrificed fit and performance by going the cheaper route. To avoid more costs, many patients skip fitting and follow-up. But these two steps actually matter more than the brand or model of hearing aid.

The trial period is also a source of problems. It's supposed to ensure patients can get a refund if the hearing aids don't meet their needs. The hearing aid manufacturers want to ensure the trial period is comfortable for the patient. Whether it actually restores hearing properly is a secondary concern. If you don't return the device within the trial period with a complaint, the dispenser and the manufacturer are happy to keep your money.

To ensure the patient's comfort on the day of sale, the hearing care provider plugs the patient's hearing test into the manufacturer's algorithm. This is what sets the amount of volume for that particular patient. Each manufacturer's algorithm automatically sets the volume lower than is required so the patient is comfortable – even though it's not the correct volume for optimum hearing. Most hearing care providers don't know this. And the only thing a person with hearing loss can assess is whether it's comfortable and whether it's better than no hearing aid at all.

Most hearing care providers don't know this. And the only thing a person with hearing loss can assess is whether it's comfortable and whether it's better than no hearing aid at all.

Why do manufacturers do this? Because someone with hearing loss has a difficult time processing sounds when they first get hearing aids. In a very real

> "Each hearing aid manufacturer's algorithm automatically sets the volume lower than is required so the patient is comfortable - even though it's not the correct volume for optimum hearing."

way, they're out of practice. Their brain hasn't had to make sense of those sounds in a long time. This is why patients with new hearing aids complain that they're too loud.

What happens after the trial period? The patient adjusts to the new sounds. They decide the change in their hearing is a hearing *problem*—and the hearing aids must be the culprit. The devices go back in the case, and the patient is no better off.

This sales-first mentality keeps some people from getting hearing aids. It leaves others with technology that should work for them but doesn't. When that happens, it's very hard to bring a patient back. Imagine you spent thousands of dollars on a product that didn't do what it was supposed to. Would you be willing to buy another set of hearing aids?

The Best Fit For You

Only a well-trained and experienced hearing care provider is skilled enough to adjust the manufacturer's preset volume for the best results. This is what is meant by "fitting" a hearing aid—a true fitting goes beyond the manufacturer's algorithm. The provider might use the presets as a starting point, but then they'll manually make adjustments to truly match your audiogram. They'll follow that with Real Ear Measurements (we'll cover this in more detail later) to verify that the programming is accurate. A custom prescription is created for YOU.

And those listening environments you discussed? Different programs will be saved to your device that approximate what you'll need in those environments. You'll be able to choose those programs when needed. Now would you be willing to buy another set of hearing aids?

CHAPTER 2

Why Hearing Loss Matters: How Treatment Can Keep You Out of the Nursing Home

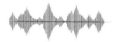

Charlie was a dedicated husband, a father to six children, and a successful and well-respected doctor. The workaholic continued to see patients into his 70s. He was particularly close to his only daughter, Kathie. They became even closer after his wife of 40 years passed away.

But Kathie started to notice a change in Charlie. It wasn't his grief over the loss of his wife. He seemed hard of hearing, and it became a running joke in the family: "Dad, didn't you hear me call you for dinner? You need hearing aids!" Charlie would typically respond, "It's not me! You guys can't expect me to hear you from another room!" or "I'll answer when I hear something interesting." Like many health care providers, however, Charlie neglected his own health.

This went on for years. Charlie would forget appointments or dinner plans, and Kathie brush it off as dad not paying attention. Until Kathie started to notice things she couldn't ignore, like when he'd forget his own address or the name of a close friend. Then a neighbor called—Charlie was there looking for his wife.

She took her dad to the doctor, where he received a battery of tests. The doctor asked her if she knew Charlie had significant hearing loss. She admitted she'd suspected it for years. What the doctor said next, though, floored her. "Did you know scientific studies show hearing loss can lead to early-onset dementia and Alzheimer's?" Her immediate thought was, "If only we'd treated Dad's hearing loss sooner, I might not be having this conversation here today."

Charlie did get hearing aids, but the damage was already done. Eventually, Kathie made the painful but necessary decision to put him in a nursing home, where he'd receive round the clock care. Kathie was crushed—her dad's twilight years wouldn't be spent in better health surrounded by family and friends.

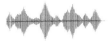

"It is not the voice that commands the story: it is the ear."
~Italo Calvino

As recently as a generation ago, most people didn't see hearing loss as a medical problem. It was thought of as a natural result of aging, a simple loss of one of the senses. It wasn't considered the serious condition that it is. I can't tell you how many conversations I've had with patients that went something like this:

Patient: "Why should I get my hearing treated?"
Me: "Well, you know your hearing loss annoys your spouse and
    family, and it affects your ability to communicate."
Patient: "I don't care if anyone can communicate with me. That's
    their problem, not mine."

Obviously, denial causes some of the prickliness. But so does our culture's general misunderstanding of the effects of hearing loss. On one hand, it's simply hearing less. But from a health perspective, hearing loss has a much more complicated and comprehensive impact. This makes sense, because it is an emotional and psychological experience, not just a sensory one.

Hearing Loss Can Shrink Your Brain… For Real

"Brain scans show us that hearing loss may contribute to a faster rate of atrophy in the brain," notes Frank Lin, Director of the Cochlear Center for Hearing and Public Health at Johns Hopkins Bloomberg School of Public Health. "Hearing loss also contributes to social isolation. You may not want to be with people as much, and when you are you may not engage in conversation as much. These factors may contribute to dementia."

Studies from across the medical community confirm Dr. Lin's hypothesis. In 2017, medical journal *The Lancet* said treating hearing loss is one of our greatest opportunities to slow down or prevent dementia. The World Health Organization (WHO) estimates that health complications from untreated hearing loss cost the world about $750 billion dollars per year.

The Lancet's 2017 Commission on Dementia Prevention, Intervention and Care presented results on modifiable risk factors for dementia (see figure below). A risk factor is something that increases the likelihood of getting a disease or injury. Removing the risk factor should, in theory, reduce the risk. **The following percentages are the potential decrease in the risk of dementia if the factor is eliminated.** For example, eliminating smoking leads to a 5% reduction in dementia risk; depression, 4%; high blood pressure, 2%; and diabetes, 1%. **The modifiable risk factor associated with the biggest decrease in risk of dementia is hearing loss, with 9%.** This is a very compelling reason for hearing loss to be a better-treated disease!

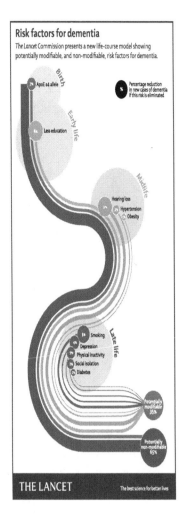

A 2019 literature review in the *Journal of the American Medical Association* found that age-related hearing loss and cognitive impairment are somehow linked. There are several possible explanations for this. It could be that one health problem—for example, blocked or reduced blood flow—leads to both conditions. Another possibility is that cognitive decline leads to hearing loss. A third possibility is that hearing loss makes the brain work harder to understand sounds, leaving less brainpower for other cognitive functions such as memory. Finally, another possibility is that the sensory deprivation of hearing loss causes the brain to become reorganized, resulting in cognitive decline.

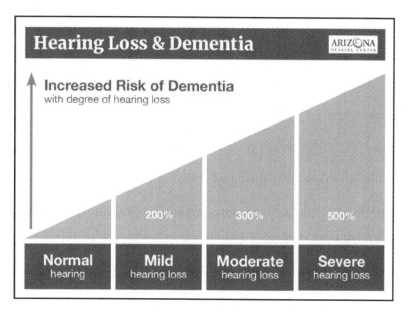

Hearing Loss Is Bad for Your Mental Health

Hearing loss can create mental health issues, even in people who've never experienced depression or anxiety. In fact, a 2018 study in *The Journal of Public Health* uncovered a link between hearing impairment and multiple mental health conditions. "We would hope those who experience hearing loss—or those living with persons who experience hearing loss—are more alert to its potential effects and better able to make informed choices about seeking help," the study's authors say.

Hearing, then, is much more than physiologically responding to sound. As Helen Keller once said, "Blindness separates us from things, but deafness separates us from people."

Think about the power of that statement for a second. When we lose the ability to hear, we lose our ability to interact with the world around us. People who've been deaf since birth are surrounded by communities who can help them. But people who experience hearing loss later in life are ill-equipped to navigate the world without the use of their ears. How does the hearing loss lead to social isolation? One conversation at a time. You don't wake up one day and suddenly feel like everyone around you is speaking gibberish. The process is a gradual one, subtle at first and eventually all-consuming. The symptoms of hearing loss manifest in myriad places, from the obvious to the unexpected. If you're not trained to see them, it's easy to miss them entirely.

> "How does hearing loss lead to social isolation? One conversation at a time. You don't wake up one day and suddenly feel like everyone around you is speaking gibberish. The process is a gradual one."

The symptoms of hearing loss manifest in myriad places, from the obvious to the unexpected. Subtle at first and eventually all-consuming. If you're not trained to see them, it's easy to miss them entirely.

Symptoms can be positive or negative. A positive symptom is something that wasn't present in your experience, and then it was. You *notice* positive symptoms, such as chest pain, shortness of breath, joint stiffness, and tinnitus. Negative symptoms are the opposite. Something has been removed from your experience, often with no clear sign it's gone. A person with hearing loss doesn't know they didn't hear something. They're often unaware of the problem and deny having a hearing loss. This makes detection very challenging.

People in the early stages of hearing loss tend to enjoy watching news, sports, and reality TV far more frequently than sitcoms or dramas. The latter genres rely far more on fast-paced dialogue and speech, which isn't helpful to viewers with hearing loss. How many context clues tell you what's happening in a scene of *Seinfeld*? It's just four people sitting in an apartment or diner chatting. Background music and laugh tracks make things even worse. As hearing loss worsens, these types of shows become harder to watch. Eventually, they're not watched at all.

But news usually features one person talking or yelling at a time. A wealth of information surrounds them to provide context. Often in reality TV, even well-hearing people can't parse what the on-screen personalities are saying. **But there are also interviews throughout in which the characters explain exactly what's going on.** Programs like *Antiques Roadshow* and *American Pickers* are popular with older demographics not just because they're nostalgic. They also clearly present the basic relevant information on screen. You might not catch everything an appraiser says, but you can see the item's name and value right before your eyes.

I bring up these examples not because watching TV is one of life's great joys—though the success of various streaming services shows it probably is—but because it shows the subtle ways hearing loss begins to sap us of our quality of life. Any hobby or pursuit that involves hearing has a similar limiting effect. People who suffer from hearing loss play fewer sports, travel to fewer places, and participate in fewer activities.

The Incredible Shrinking World Of Hearing Loss

That's why people with hearing loss live in a world that's growing ever smaller. The planet remains the same size; their access to it does not. People with hearing loss slowly begin to feel like strangers in their own environments. The entire world can seem like a foreign country. If you've ever traveled overseas and don't speak the language, you know how the local culture is closed off to you.

People with hearing loss experience a growing feeling of alienation that follows a pattern. First, they stop going to restaurants and similar places. It's just too frustrating trying to communicate amid background noise. Then, they stop interacting with strangers altogether. Even ordering a coffee becomes an arduous task. After that, they spend less time with friends and acquaintances, offering excuses like "I don't like socializing anyway" or "There are a lot of things I don't want to hear." Finally, only their closest relatives are willing to put in the effort and patience required to carry on even a simple conversation. When the family gathers, the person with hearing loss sits in silence. They may have plenty to say, but they can't follow the conversation. The essence of humanity is relationships. Hearing loss slowly takes this away.

I'd Like to Teach the World To Hear In Perfect Harmony

And of course, there's music. Neurologist Oliver Sacks, one of the best-loved scientists of the 20th century, wrote an entire book dedicated to the incredible impact music has on our brains: *Musicophilia: Tales of Music and the Brain*. In it, he quotes Schopenhauer:

"The inexpressible depth of music, so easy to understand and yet so inexplicable, is due to the fact that it reproduces all the emotions of our innermost being, but entirely without reality and remote from its pain....Music expresses only the quintessence of life and of its events, never these themselves."

Missing out on these depths of beauty, especially when we have the ability to prevent that absence, is tragic. You'll remember my grandfather, the bandleader, who taught me early on about the power and beauty of music. He would certainly view it as a tragedy if hearing loss limited his ability to experience the depth and quality and nuances of music.

Why We Don't Act Fast Enough

Waiting until communication fails is far too late to begin treating hearing loss. The second you notice a loved one asking "What?" a little too regularly or more than once to the same question, it's time to schedule an appointment. Ideally, you should get a full audiological evaluation by the time you turn 60. Like other degenerative conditions, the sooner hearing loss is detected, the easier it is to remedy. The only way to truly detect hearing loss is with a professional evaluation.

> "Waiting until communication fails is far too late to begin treating hearing loss. The second you notice a loved one asking 'What?' a little too regularly, it's time to schedule an appointment."

Perhaps the easiest way to illustrate the importance of early treatment is by comparison. How long would you wait to get glasses or contact lenses? Would you do something when you first noticed vision problems, or would you wait until you can't see well enough to drive your car? The answer is clear, even if your vision isn't.

For some reason, hearing aids carry a stigma that glasses don't, even though one could argue that hearing loss is even more impactful on our lives than visual impairment. My saying this is in no way similar to the sophomoric bar conversation about whether you'd rather be deaf or blind. Neither is desirable, and to ask that question or compare the two in that way is offensive to both vision- and hearing-impaired people. I do find it curious, though, that hearing aids carry a huge stigma that glasses don't.

Rebecca Rosen interviewed artist and engineer Sarah Hendren for *The Atlantic*. Hendren speculated the stigma may be in part because we consider hearing aids "assistive technology"—a way to bring someone up to speed with the world, much like a wheelchair does. She asserts this way of thinking only leads to us limiting ourselves. "By returning 'assistive technology' to its rightful place as just 'technology'—no more, no less—we start to understand that all bodies are getting assistance, all the time," she writes.

This distinction is crucial, because it reconfigures our perception of hearing aids. Right now, you might be wearing a watch that monitors your heart rate. Odds are you have a phone that tracks your steps. We don't view these devices as compensation for our own failings. We don't think of glasses as a sign of weakness. Hearing aids, for any number of reasons, are not accepted the same way.

The True Scope Of Hearing Loss

Treating hearing loss early and effectively is critical. It affects our lives in unnoticed ways until we've fallen into the abyss of hearing loss. It changes the way we interact in the world and the happiness we get from daily life. That's a huge deal.

> *Healthy, robust hearing is about music. It's about laughter. It's about stories. It's about conversation. It's about friends, and family and relationships. It's about your ability to think, remember, and understand. It is, in short, about the very things that make life worth living. And that, more than anything, is why treating hearing loss early and effectively really matters.*

CHAPTER 3

Communication Problems vs. Hearing Loss

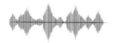

Nicknamed "The King," Arnold Palmer is known as one of the greatest and most dynamic professional golfers of all time. In a career spanning more than six decades, he won 62 PGA Tour titles and was inducted into the World Golf Hall of Fame. A charismatic man, few know that he suffered from gradual hearing loss for more than 30 years.

Palmer said that without hearing aids he couldn't understand what most people said to him. Jim Blasingame wrote of him after his passing: "When you saw Arnold deliver his patented thumbs-up response with those massive hands, that was his way of coping with the fact that he heard someone addressing him, but didn't hear what was said. It was troubling to me that someone might think he was being arrogant or dismissive by not answering, when nothing could be further from the truth."

Palmer himself acknowledged that he wore two hearing aids to improve his communication and understanding. In an interview with Dr. Douglas Beck for Healthy Hearing, he said: "There was a time when I couldn't hear what most people said to me, most of the time. But with the hearing aids, I understand just about everything. So probably if I had to identify one primary issue—it would be conversational speech, and I have to tell you the quality of the sound is so nice now—it really is very impressive." The hearing aids made it so he could function in a crowded room without having to give his thumbs-up sign or ask others to speak up. He knew that to stay connected to the world around him, he needed to keep up with advances in hearing technology.

But perhaps the biggest bonus of good hearing for Palmer involved his golf game. In that same interview with Dr. Beck, he said, "I think that when I hear myself better, when I can better monitor how my voice sounds, I can do a better job speaking. And VERY importantly, better hearing has made a difference in my golf game! ... I've noticed the sound of the golf ball being hit by the golf club is different, and much more realistic, with the hearing aids. The sound with the hearing aids makes sense, and better represents what I know is happening to the golf ball."

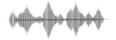

Golf legend Arnold Palmer's experience demonstrates how hearing loss hinders everyday communication. That's a given. It also highlights the problem—we've decided hearing loss is only real when it interferes with communication. Mr. Palmer's hearing loss story occurred more than 15 years ago and yet, people are still reluctant to treat their hearing loss at the early signs of trouble.

A patient has hearing loss long before it seeps into everyday conversations. Sure, having difficulty with verbal communication is a symptom. But there are ways to scientifically measure the presence of hearing loss long before communication falters. Unfortunately, patients often don't recognize the early stages—they don't know what they're not hearing. I suspect Mr. Palmer's hearing loss affected his awareness of how he connected with the golf ball long before he was aware of his hearing loss.

There are many reasons people don't recognize the early stages of hearing loss. For one, most varieties of hearing loss are progressive, including age-related hearing loss. You don't wake up one morning with everything on mute as though you're starring in your own silent movie. Instead, ranges of sounds gradually disappear from your life, with higher pitches dropping out first. Arnold Palmer constantly adapted new technology to address his needs over the 30 years he experienced progressive hearing loss.

You can go on YouTube right now and search "How Old Are Your Ears?" to experience the progressive hearing loss phenomenon for yourself. As of this writing, the video has nearly 20 million views, so it's clearly a popular activity.

Rudimentary tests like these are fun but impractical. The range of frequencies used and the way they are applied does not represent real-world hearing. Later in this book, we'll discuss in detail how audiograms and other tests can empirically and comprehensively screen for hearing loss well before it affects communication. This chapter, though, focuses on how hearing loss impacts communication and how our brains allow us to communicate long after hearing loss is present.

The Music Gets Softer

If you've ever invested in a nice pair of headphones or speakers, you know what a difference good audio equipment makes. You pick up lots of nuances you simply wouldn't hear over your laptop or phone's built-in speakers. You experience a familiar song in a different way that's hard to describe. If you never hear the enhanced version, you may not even realize what you're missing. But comparing one to the other proves a stark difference. When given the choice, you'd always rather have the hi-fi sound.

Progressive hearing loss is like going from hi-fi to low-quality speakers slowly. The change is gradual, so it's impossible to perceive the difference. Again, you don't know what you can't hear. Because the structure of the song remains the same, your experience *feels* the same. In a very demonstrable way, though, your experience is actually much worse.

Another useful analogy to explain this phenomenon is weight gain. How does somebody gain too much weight? One ounce at a time. You're not 200 pounds one week and by the next week 500 pounds. Hearing loss works the same way, but it's sneakier. As your hearing begins to fail, you don't have an easy reference point, like you do with pants size. Your brain wants you to communicate and understand, and it will allow you to do so long after hearing loss is noticeable.

These comparisons are helpful, but how hearing loss progressively interferes with speech comprehension is a much trickier matter. Communication is a two-way street, and we're used to driving on it. At first, we can subconsciously infer the sounds we don't hear. Eventually, however, too many sounds go missing. The brain can't compensate. Usually, a patient and their loved ones wait to reckon with hearing loss until after this process is well underway. By then, what I like to call The *Wheel of Fortune* Effect has begun.

You Can't Buy A Consonant

Fundamental to the game show *Wheel of Fortune* is the rule that you have to buy a vowel—as long as you can afford one—but you have to spin the wheel to guess a consonant. Why is this distinction so integral to the show?

Because consonants give words meaning. A contestant can buy all five vowels as quickly as possible and still be no closer to solving the puzzle. If they guess the right combination of key consonants, however, they might figure out the solution with just a few guesses.

Don't believe me? Here's an actual *Wheel of Fortune* puzzle with just the vowels. The category, since you'd be given that on the show, is Thing.

$$\_\ O\ U\ \_\ \_$$
$$\_\ O\ \_\ \_\ O\ U\ \_$$

Any guesses? Pretty tough, right? If that seems like an unfair puzzle to solve, look how easy it becomes when you have all the consonants instead.

$$T\ \_\ \_\ GH$$
$$W\ \_\ RK\ \_\ \_\ T$$

The difference is stark, and that's because of the way language—it's true of the vast majority of world languages, not just English—is structured around consonants. As the poet Samuel Taylor Coleridge once wrote, "[A]nimals have the vowel sounds; man alone can utter consonants."

These consonant sounds, which are the first to go, are the most essential for being able to communicate effectively. Imagine your life becoming a game of *Wheel of Fortune* that gets a little bit harder every day, until eventually you're left with only vowels. That's how hearing loss operates.

Some patients, as they lose consonants, tell me, "I know people are talking to me, but I can't understand what they're saying."

"Imagine your life becoming a game of *Wheel of Fortune* that gets a little bit harder every day, until eventually you're left with only vowels. That's how hearing loss operates."

However, as with every other type of sound, consonants don't disappear in one fell swoop. Parts of sounds get worn down gradually until they're gone altogether. Their near-total disintegration often goes unnoticed. Furthermore, the brain knows how important speech comprehension is. It has a toolset for piecing sound fragments together into coherent words. And it can do this far longer than you might expect. The puzzle can be completed, as it were, even when a good number of pieces are missing.

The Myth Of Situational Hearing Loss

Hearing loss is tricky in another way. It makes people think they only have trouble hearing in certain situations. Scientifically, this claim is simply not true. Environment is irrelevant. If you have hearing loss in a crowded restaurant, you just as surely have it when you're at home. However, I totally understand why people seem to only experience their hearing loss in certain situations.

Hearing, for all intents and purposes, doesn't work in a vacuum. The sensation of listening is actually the result of three distinct processes working together. Imagine a three-legged stool. One leg is the auditory process of hearing, another is speech-reading, and the third is speech context. The auditory process is the biological component—the ears, auditory nerve, and brain. Speech-reading is all the nonverbal cues, from lip-reading to gestures to facial animation. Speech context includes the setting a conversation happens in as well as the words before and after a given set of sounds. Language and communication, as most people experience them, require all three legs of the stool to function properly.

Because the three legs of the stool work in concert, you have a lifetime of experience associating each leg with the other two. When one of them falters, you instinctively prop it up with the other two. Sometimes, this compensating is conscious. For example, if you're on the phone, you can't rely on speech-reading, so you focus more on the person's voice. The buffoon wandering into traffic while talking on the phone is a cliché for a reason: Ignoring your surroundings does make it easier to hear the person on the other end of the phone.

THE THREE LEGGED STOOL OF COMMUNICATION

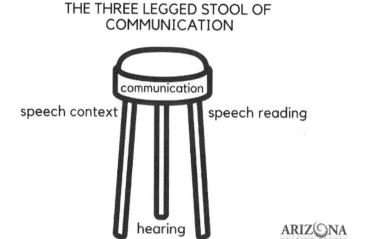

Sometimes, the compensation process kicks in unnoticed, as in the early stage of hearing loss. As one leg of the stool, the hearing gradually weakens, the two remaining strong legs pick up the slack. In the early stages of hearing loss, when a person says they have a hearing loss in certain situations, it actually means one of the other two legs of the stool is being restricted. It isn't situational hearing loss—it means either speech-reading or speech context is having trouble compensating. The result is you notice that your hearing is failing.

Compensations In Action

Sometimes my patients bristle at the suggestion that they're speech-reading. "I don't know how to read lips," they say. You're probably not a trained lip-reader, but you can absolutely read lips to some extent. It's baked into the cognitive wiring of anyone born with both sight and sound. You use mouth movements to confirm what you're hearing, and vice versa. That's why it's so irritating to watch a video where the sound and image don't sync up. Your brain expects a mouth to make particular movements when it emits particular sounds. You can instantly tell when something is amiss.

Once this connection between sound and movement is hardwired into the brain, it doesn't go away. As hearing loss occurs, you rely on these associations to pick up the slack. Even if you're not aware of it, your brain associates certain sounds with certain mouth movements, allowing you to intuit sounds you can't actually hear.

This is especially true with the people closest to you. You've watched your spouse's mouth sound out a near-infinite number of

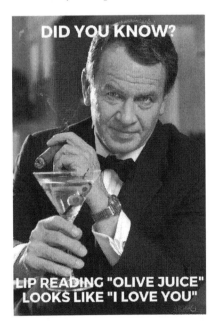

words over the years. They can probably relay a message to you across a crowded room without you hearing them. Think about how many times you got the message when your partner mouthed the words "I love you." See? You can lip-read.

Your English teachers told you that if you didn't understand the meaning of a word, you could use context clues to guess before consulting a dictionary. You do the same thing when you

34

don't hear a word perfectly. Nobody thinks their spouse is asking them to "map the floors," even if that's what it sounds like.

These compensation methods are not learned skills present only in patients who've cultivated them, they're built-in mechanisms designed to function exactly as they do. Their evolutionary benefit is clear: Long before hearing loss was treatable, people needed to compensate for its early stages. We are hardwired to put off its negative effects for as long as possible. Now that we have the option to treat hearing loss, our defense tactics actually work against us. They fool us into thinking we're fine when we're really not.

The bottom line is that communication problems are not the same thing as hearing loss. If you wait for the former to be a regular issue before treating the latter, you've already waited too long.

Stop Guessing, Start Knowing

It's maddening that we don't treat hearing testing the same way we do so many other types of medical screening. We don't wait until a patient starts complaining to

"The National Institute on Deafness and Other Communication Disorders estimates that about 30-35% of adults ages 65+ suffer from hearing loss. For adults ages 75+, that number jumps to 40-50%."

screen for colorectal cancer, and we shouldn't do it for hearing loss, either. Every patient deserves to know as early as possible if they have hearing loss. This should be an easy win – yet we don't do it.

The National Institute on Deafness and Other Communication Disorders estimates that about 30%-35% of adults ages 65 and older suffer from hearing loss. For adults ages 75 and older, that number jumps to 40%-50%. We should be testing for it annually.

Treating hearing loss will become more commonplace when hearing testing becomes more commonplace. The biggest obstacle is the 1:1 link we've created between hearing loss and communication problems. We must treat communication issues as a sign of late-stage hearing loss, not the first alarm bells of trouble. The alternative is a more isolated existence cut off from joyful life experiences as well as increased risk for early dementia and Alzheimer's disease (I discuss this more fully in a later chapter). Early testing for hearing loss seems like a relatively easy step to prevent problems down the road.

The Message Is Clear

Get your hearing tested. Don't speculate about whether you have hearing loss. Don't wait for communication to become a chore. Find out for sure as early as possible. If you're over 60, ask about a hearing evaluation at your next doctor's appointment. As with so many other conditions, early detection of hearing loss gives you a wider variety of treatment options.

CHAPTER 4

Hearing Loss Impacts Everyone—
Deal With It

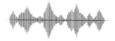

Cindy is extremely close to her daughters. She's devoted to their happiness and wants nothing but the best for them. A single mom, she even recently moved to a different state to be close to them and her grandchildren. Cindy spends her time and talents renovating and decorating her daughters' homes and shuttling her grandchildren to their various activities. Positive and outgoing, her beautiful smile lights up the room at any gathering.

But she also suffers from progressive hearing loss. Cindy knows it, and others notice that she becomes quiet in large social gatherings. Like many things in her life, though, she sees her hearing loss as her burden to bear alone. Cindy thinks it only impacts her, so she doesn't feel the need for a hearing test. She'd rather just cope, as she has with so many other challenges, because she thinks she's doing just fine without hearing aids.

Her well-intentioned and self-sacrificing course of action fails to recognize how hearing loss impacts those around her. Cindy often asks her daughters multiple times to repeat directions to the grandchildren's school. Often when Cindy offers to do the grocery shopping, she misses a few things the kids asked her to pick up. Though her daughters are inconvenienced by these lapses, they're more concerned about Cindy's well being. They want her to enjoy a full and beautiful life that matches her beautiful smile.

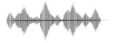

What We Get Wrong About Hearing Loss

There are many myths and misconceptions about hearing loss. Often, they're perpetuated by those who experience hearing loss as well as by those living with them.

"It Only Affects Me"

The most common myth I hear from my patients is that their hearing loss only affects them. Trying to put an end to any conversation about treatment, they'll say, "I'm doing just fine." (Based on my conversations with general physicians, I'd say they hear that excuse even more than I do. When you've already been referred to an ear specialist like me, after all, it's harder to feign ignorance.) The patient places the burden of hearing loss squarely on their own shoulders, assuming that leaves them free to solve the problem as they see fit. "If hearing loss only hurts me," the reasoning goes, "then it's up to me to decide if and when I want to treat it."

The problem here? This just isn't true. It might be your hearing that's failing, but your hearing loss affects everyone around you. For example, it's common for people with minor to moderate hearing loss to rely on their spouse to interact with the rest of the world. Suppose, then, that I have hearing loss. If my wife needs to order meals at a restaurant for me, that's a qualitative change in her life. She doesn't have hearing loss, but she is absolutely affected by mine.

Getting treated for hearing loss, then, is also about everyone who cares for and interacts with me as well.

"I Hear Better Than…"

Another myth I hear from my patients is similar to this: "My hearing is better than so-and-so's. They don't have hearing aids, so I'm fine." As with the last myth, this simply isn't true, and it's definitely not helpful. True, the effects of hearing loss are social, but the condition isn't measured by how well those around you can hear. The only meaningful way to measure it is by comparing what you can hear to what you should be able to hear. As mentioned before, there are ways to scientifically detect hearing loss well before communication problems arise. A patient simply is not the best judge of their own hearing ability.

"Hearing Loss Isn't A Health Condition"

The final myth is one I touched on earlier, and it's a dangerous one: Hearing loss is not a health condition. An earlier chapter has ample evidence disproving this argument. Hearing loss can negatively impact your mental and physical health. The idea that it's only a problem with one of your five senses needs to be thrown in the trash.

Needed: An Up-to-Date Perspective

These misconceptions perpetuate wrong-headed thinking. They also prevent an up-to-date and productive perspective on hearing loss. If we can't accurately discuss the issue, how are we supposed to solve it? Some of our failings are historical, others cultural, and still others have no logical origin whatsoever. But they all get the fundamental essence of hearing loss wrong.

Just as the way we test for and treat hearing loss is in need of an urgent upgrade, so too is the way we talk about hearing loss. We've locked ourselves into a series of stock clichés that are heavy on excuses but light on solutions. We've let outdated ideas persist for decades. In short, we've created a conversation that doesn't serve its purpose. It's high time we rectify that.

What Hearing Aids Have in Common With Assisted Living

How we talk about hearing aids is even worse than how we talk about hearing loss. Many of us buy a new phone every year—why do we still think hearing aids look like they did in the 1980s? Newsflash: Hearing technology has advanced just as much as any other type of tech. Nobody buys a gigantic, brick-shaped cell phone anymore, and the same can be said of hearing aids.

Here, again, that interview with Sarah Hendren in *The Atlantic* is relevant. Glasses, Hendren suggests, are not considered a tool for people who are "handicapped" or in need of "assistive technology." For some reason, though, hearing aids have not escaped this stigma. Patients often see a hearing aid as a serious disruption to their life. She argues that all technology is assistive by nature. Stigmatizing technology keeps people from confidently seeking it out. "By returning 'assistive technology' to its rightful place as just 'technology'—no more, no less—we start to understand that all bodies are getting assistance, all the time," she writes. That's exactly what needs to happen with hearing aids.

Getting a hearing aid leads to a negligible cosmetic difference— not getting one can reshape your entire life. Hearing loss is like baseball, but worse, because you only get two strikes with hearing loss. Ask somebody to repeat something one time, and you're fine. If you need to ask a second time, they'll probably give up. The usual answer to the second "What?" is "Never mind."

That might sound harsh, but it's true. Nobody wants to repeat something to you over and over again. Your loved ones might put up with it, but the barista at the coffee shop will regard you

"Hearing loss is like baseball, but worse, because you only get two strikes with hearing loss. Ask somebody to repeat something one time, and you're fine. If you need to ask again, they'll probably say 'never mind'."

with contempt in a hurry. Isn't that a bigger disturbance than having hearing aids?

Since Rosen wrote her article, our society has embraced tech to an even greater degree. Walk the streets in a major city today and you'll see dozens of people with AirPods hanging from their ears. These headphones are far more conspicuous than modern hearing aids, but they're not considered a sign of weakness or degradation. They're just the opposite. Wearing them comes with a sense of prestige and cultural cachet. Hearing aids needn't be any different, provided we escape the brick-phone mentality that persists.

Which brings us to assisted-living facilities. There was a time when the elderly in the U.S. feared being moved out of the family home because it meant going to live in a dismal and gloomy nursing home. That image has persisted; so older Americans today tend to be understandably resistant to leaving their family home. Such accommodations are seen as a personal affront at best and a complete abandonment at worst.

In the first season of *The Sopranos*, Tony Soprano struggles to convince his mother, Livia, to move into a lavish facility that more closely resembles a resort at Cap d'Antibes than a stereotypical nursing home. "Green Grove is a retirement community," Tony pleads with his mother, but the message never gets through.

Both of these ideas—that hearing aids are visibly obtrusive and that nursing homes are miserable places—are outdated, but we use them as crutches to avoid having difficult conversations. Fortunately, the younger generations recognize that technology can improve quality of life. I hope the current 50-year-olds who love Facebook become 70-year-olds who embrace wearing a device that makes life richer and more enjoyable. To accomplish that, however, there's one mental obstacle we need to put to the sword—vanity.

The Vanity Excuse Is BS

"Oh, my grandmother is too vain to get a hearing aid."

This is the most common type of excuse I hear from family members. You know who I never hear this from? Patients. Most don't have any deep-seated qualms about hearing aids. They might have minor protests, but nothing that sound reasoning and a caring approach can't overcome.

The vanity excuse protects loved ones, not patients. Claiming Grandma is vain is a dodge. It absolves loved ones (in their minds) of the responsibility to help Grandma live a fuller and more meaningful life. It proves they made nominal effort to get the treatment process started, and it failed because of the incurable reason of vanity. Here, as with the "my hearing loss, my decision" line of thinking, a dead end is created when there shouldn't be one.

If you have a loved one with hearing loss, they will be receptive to discussing it if your approach is open and honest. "I don't want a hearing aid" is not the end of a conversation—it's the beginning. You have to be willing to talk about how their hearing loss affects you if you want them to take it seriously. You could even make an appointment for yourself, then bring the person who actually needs treatment with you. The faster you can make the matter medical, not personal, the quicker you'll conquer their misgivings.

I Do Not Want Hearing Aids

When I tell patients they need appropriately selected, well-fitted hearing aids to treat their hearing loss, the standard response is simply, "I do not want hearing aids." This response isn't surprising, given the common misperceptions about hearing loss and hearing aids. No one *wants* hearing aids. Some who *need* hearing aids do pursue the technology and experience the benefits.

There are very few health issues that lead to patients wanting the prescribed treatment. The treatment is taken with the expectation of improvement. Someone takes

> "Someone with hearing loss doesn't get hearing aids only for themselves - hearing aids are for everyone else. They enable hearing loss sufferers to better connect with loved ones, family, friends, and society!"

blood pressure medication every morning to lower their blood pressure. Someone gets a vaccine to ensure immunity. Certainly, very few people *like* medicine or shots.

Here's an extreme example. A person who has the misfortune of losing a leg has options for their rehabilitation—hop on one leg, use a crutch, or be fitted for a prosthetic leg. None of these options reverses the loss of a leg. However, each option restores mobility to a lesser or greater extent. What if you saw a person hopping on one leg? It would seem absurd, and you would wonder why they didn't get a prosthetic leg or, at the very least, a crutch.

For some reason, people don't see hearing loss in the same way. A person with untreated hearing loss might as well be hopping on one leg. The rehabilitation only works if one uses it. "I do not want hearing aids" misses the point. Someone with hearing loss doesn't get hearing aids only for themselves – hearing aids are for everyone else. They enable hearing loss sufferers to better connect with loved ones, family, friends, and society!

How To Speak To Someone With Hearing Loss

Not everyone with hearing loss gets it treated in a timely fashion. Indeed, if they did, I wouldn't have to write this book. There's a large gap between the prevalence of hearing loss and its treatment. This means you probably have a friend or family member who lives with hearing loss. Communicating with these folks is often a taxing experience. You know what you want to express, but not how to do so effectively. They want to understand, but they don't know how to coach you in what they need to do so. You're both mentally capable of holding a conversation, but there's an auditory barrier to successful communication.

Speaking with somebody who has hearing loss will always involve a little friction. However, you can make it a little smoother. At my practice, Arizona Hearing Center, we provide patients and their loved ones with 18 tips that help bridge the gap between the fully hearing and the hearing impaired.

Some of the tips are:

- Do not shout. Increasing your volume might distort what you're saying.
- Listeners often rely on speech-reading to compensate for hearing loss. Speech-reading is using lip-reading, facial expressions, and gestures to understand a conversation.
- Multiple conversations are a more challenging listening environment. Conversing with four or fewer people usually results in one person speaking at a time. With five or more people, the result is usually at least two conversations.
- The listener should avoid saying "I didn't hear you" or "What?" This prompts the speaker to say the same thing more

loudly, which doesn't help. Instead, they should say, "I didn't understand you." The speaker can then express the same thought in a different way. This encourages understanding because the same information is said differently.

*Visit **ListenUpHearing.com/register** to receive our 18 Tips for Speaking to People with Hearing Loss.*

With these tips, you can make conversations with hearing-impaired people easier, but tips are no substitute for treating hearing loss. Until we live in a world where everyone who needs hearing loss treatment receives it, these tools will be useful. But they'll never be a perfect solution.

CHAPTER 5

Why Selling Hearing Aids Is The Wrong Mindset

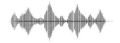

After years of gentle nagging by her daughter, Betsy, Janet finally decided she would consider buying hearing aids. She'd seen plenty of hearing aid advertisements over the years, but she really liked a commercial that often aired during the news: A grandfather celebrates getting "low-cost hearing aids" and complains about doctors gouging patients by charging "anything they want." Janet, like many folks, thought of hearing aids as a commodity—you price shop and get the cheapest pair. She told her daughter, "I don't want to break the bank. Just find me something that doesn't cost too much."

An online search for low-cost and discount hearing aids directed them to the local Costco, which sold hearing aids on site. The website emphasized "value pricing" and had the word "free" everywhere—free product demonstrations, free hearing tests, free appointments, free loss and damage coverage, free warranties, free follow-up. Free, free, free! Janet was happy with that, so off they went.

A very nice young lady checked Janet's hearing and gave her some hearing aids. They seemed to work for the first couple of months. But the initial enthusiasm of hearing certain sounds again wore off. She noticed sounds were too loud. There was a buzzing in her ears. She stopped putting her hearing aids in each morning. Eventually, the hearing aids—which were supposed to solve her problem—spent more time in a drawer than in her ears. She never went back to Costco to have them checked. She assumed she was one of those patients that hearing aids couldn't help.

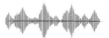

We Don't Sell Hearing Aids. We Treat Hearing Loss.

Those two sentences are the crux of my approach. They are the purest essence of my position as a care provider and physician. They are the surest route to fixing our dysfunctional hearing care system. Technically speaking, we do sell hearing aids—you can procure from us a technological solution to your hearing loss. But saying we "sell" a product misses the point entirely.

Saying we don't sell hearing aids can throw patients for a loop, but it serves a purpose. I don't want my patients to see hearing aids as simply a product to buy. For nearly as long as hearing aids have existed, they've been treated as a commodity no different than a TV or a roll of toilet paper. But these commoditized hearing aids often don't work properly. Everything's too loud, or the hearing aids are very uncomfortable.

If a hearing aid isn't appropriately selected and adjusted by a knowledgeable provider who understands your personal hearing health needs, it won't serve its intended purpose—treating hearing loss.

Commodity vs. Service

Commodity

When a solution is commoditized, the purchaser expects it to solve a problem right away once purchased. With the receipt in hand, the work is done. Sure, it might have to be set up a tad—formatting a new iPhone or throwing some steaks on a grill—but the transaction is the hard part.

Approaching hearing aids this same way is a recipe for disaster. You don't buy a hearing aid, stick it in your ear, and call it a day. A hearing aid is not a magic pill that solves all your problems. It works after being tailored to the unique nature of your specific hearing loss and the needs of your listening environment. It's also part of a suite of treatment services that allows you to function despite hearing loss.

Service

As a patient, you can only tell if your hearing aid works better than nothing at all. To find out if it works as well as it should, you need guided testing. To understand why, let's look at how your brain reacts to hearing technology.

When you start wearing hearing aids, your brain is presented with sounds it hasn't encountered in years. It can be overwhelming. So it's better to gradually increase the amount of information presented to your ears and brain. Follow-ups allow your provider to ensure the device is working properly and as intended.

But it's also an opportunity for you to describe the new situations you've encountered since the last visit and how your devices could handle them better. This allows your provider to make further adjustments to your programming.

To optimize the outcome of your better-hearing journey, it's essential to have an experienced professional guiding and educating you along the way. Simply put, care and treatment matter.

Which Hearing Aid Should I Buy?

This is the most common question I'm asked. I answer that the brand doesn't really matter. There is no single hearing aid manufacturer who makes the best hearing aid in each class and category.

It's just like cars. If someone asked you which company makes the best car, you would probably expect them to narrow it down to a specific type of car, such as subcompact, full-size, small SUV, luxury SUV, minivan, or a pickup truck. Why? Because no single company makes the best vehicle across all types.

Hearing aids are similar. You should be much more concerned about the expertise of the provider than what brand of hearing aid is used. A high-quality provider will stay up to date on the current technology. They'll know what's best for your hearing loss and listening lifestyle.

A Better Way

The treatment-as-commodity mindset is the most dangerous aspect of our cultural conception of hearing loss. It informs our warped discourse about the nature and treatment of hearing loss, and it's a major reason why the treatment rate hovers around 20 percent. Nobody needs to be sold on a kidney transplant—they shouldn't have to be sold on a hearing aid.

I urge you to stop regarding hearing aids as objects to buy. Think of them as one component in a comprehensive course of treating hearing loss. Maybe one day we'll have hearing technology that is completely responsive to the wearer and requires no human intervention. We're a long way off from that dream. Until then, our hearing technology will only achieve optimal performance when rigorously fitted by a professional and adjusted as needed over time. The patient needs to be guided and educated through their better-hearing journey.

> "Our hearing technology will only achieve optimal performance when rigorously fitted by a professional and adjusted as needed. Patients need to be guided and educated on their better-hearing journey."

Let's vow to stop buying and selling hearing aids. Let's start treating hearing loss as the multi-faceted and individualized condition that it is. In the next section of this book, I explain how we can do just that by using the greatest set of diagnostic and treatment tools available in human history. Whatever mistakes we have made in the past, there's nothing stopping us from creating a much brighter and more sonorous future.

CHAPTER 6

Comparison Shopping For Hearing Loss Treatment: Quality Counts

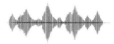

Do you remember the '80s movie The Money Pit, starring Tom Hanks? Walter (played by Hanks) and his girlfriend, Anna (played by Shelley Long), need a new home in a hurry. They settle on a multi-million dollar country estate outside New York City priced suspiciously low. They quickly discover the reason for the price as doors fall off, a bathtub falls through the floor, and the staircase collapses. And if that isn't enough, the plumbing is full of gunk, the electrical system catches on fire, and a raccoon lives in the dumbwaiter.

Walter and Anna hire some bungling contractors, who keep promising the repairs will "take two more weeks." Instead, the contractors make matters worse because they don't know what they're doing and care more about the money. The work drags on for months, the bills pile up, and the problems never get solved. As a result, the couple's relationship also falls apart.

Walter and Anna's experience is a classic buyer-beware scenario. Quite simply, if the price seems too good to be true for the promised quality, it usually is. This is true for most thing, including hearing aids.

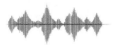

Home Repair Is Not A Commodity

Walter and Anna fell into a common consumer trap—looking for the highest quality service for the cheapest price. But in home renovation, like with most things, the two rarely go hand in hand.

It all starts with the best of intentions. After figuring out the cost of goods, you know you still need to pay for the job to get done. But three different companies using the same materials come up with wildly different estimates for you. How is that?

If you wanted to build a brick wall, you'd compare prices at the big-box home-supply retailers and buy the bricks and mortar at the best price. You wouldn't care about the brands of the materials. You'd care about price and availability. This is the typical way to purchase a commodity—price is the main motivator, not the brand.

If you have the materials delivered to your home, you still don't have a brick wall. You just have materials. You still need to hire a mason to use the brick and mortar to build the wall. You get three bids, select the middle bid, and end up finding the quality of work unacceptable. You hire the more expensive mason to either fix the poor work or rebuild the wall. Turns out, the quality of the brick wall was directly related to the skill of the mason.

What would you choose: A bad stonemason using good brick or a great stonemason using average brick? Certainly, the wall would be better from a high-quality mason. Why? The craftsmanship affects the outcome more than does the materials used. Similarly, the outcome of the hearing care is directly related to the skill of the hearing care professional.

With hearing loss treatment, you have to choose quality service over low cost. You might get the same hearing aid from two different providers, but its performance won't be the same. An audiologist fits a hearing aid to your needs just as a contractor fits materials to your project. In both cases, the service is more important than the materials themselves. If you understand this premise, it becomes a lot easier to treat your hearing loss in a way that works.

An Ideal Course Of Quality Hearing Loss Treatment

At the beginning of this book, I laid out the average American's experience when seeking out treatment for hearing loss. I discussed barriers to treatment and why treatment is often so unsuccessful. As a counterpoint, let's take a look at an optimal course of treatment.

Suppose you turn 60 and already experience moderate hearing loss. You might be referred to an ear surgeon like me. I'll ensure the problem can be treated through hearing aids rather than, for example, a good ear cleaning or surgery. If I can rule out medical intervention, I will send you for a comprehensive hearing evaluation.

The Comprehensive Evaluation

The hearing care provider will evaluate your hearing ability, but they'll also assess your listening lifestyle. Are you a business executive who actively participates in daily meetings? Or do you live in a nursing home where you only see your family once a month? Perhaps you regularly go to the theater and symphony with their friends? The recommended course of treatment will depend on your lifestyle and listening environments. Everyone is different, so everyone requires a different hearing treatment plan.

The Hearing Aid Fitting

Remember from Chapter 1 that a high-quality provider manually programs beyond the manufacturer's software. This is why understanding your listening lifestyle is key. Your provider pairs the right technology to your lifestyle, then fits it so it's custom-tailored to your needs.

Hundreds of different questions and issues can arise. This is not a solo journey. You need a highly skilled hearing care professional who will guide you as well as help you understand your hearing loss and the better-hearing process. The more educated you are about hearing loss, the more successful your journey will be. Don't be afraid to ask questions. The alternative? Investing time and money on high-quality, poorly fit hearing aids that whistle all the time.

The Trial and Adjustment Period

As mentioned in the previous chapter, during the trial period (in this case, 90 days), your ears and brain need to get used to their new hearing aids. They'll be reencountering sound that, over time, they'd grown accustomed to not hearing. Your listening lifestyle and environment are unique, but you'll also adjust to hearing technology differently from anyone else.

> "During the trial period, your ears and brain need to get used to their new hearing aids. They'll be reencountering sounds that, over time, they'd grown accustomed to not hearing."

During the adjustment process, your questions will be specific to how you're experiencing restored hearing. Sounds might be too loud. You might be hearing too much. You might be frustrated at how your hearing technology responds to different listening situations. Once the accommodation period is complete and both you *and* your provider are happy with the aids' performance, you'll wear your hearing aids all day, every day, and take good care of them.

Follow-Ups

But your journey isn't over! Your provider reexamines and interviews you about every six months to ensure the aids still match your needs and listening lifestyle. Your provider will also regularly assess you for alternative and new technology. This continues for three to five years. At that point, your devices will most likely no longer fit your needs and will need to be replaced.

That, in broad strokes, is what ideal hearing care should look like. It's completely attainable, but we're a long way from making it commonplace. Achieving this ideal is only possible when you take control of your health care and seek out the highest quality care.

How To Know If You're Getting Quality Hearing Care

The art critic and philosopher John Ruskin once said, "Quality is never an accident. It is always the result of intelligent effort." What you should seek at all stages of your treatment is intelligent effort. Somebody who tries hard isn't necessarily giving you what you need. Many of my new patients say their current hearing care provider is a nice person who tries hard and does their best. My honest answer to that is always, "Earnest incompetence is still incompetence." The problem remains untreated.

One Simple Question

With discernment, you can tell early on whether your provider is making an intelligent effort. A great way to test this is to ask a simple question right after you complete your hearing test:

Which model of hearing aid should I buy?

If your provider lists a few options, you have a right to be skeptical. If they give you a single model and say it's the one for you, run for the hills. The nature of your hearing loss and the hearing aid you need is not a 1:1 equation. There are (seriously) thousands of hearing aid models, with new ones being released all the time. A provider who claims they can select the perfect one for you based on the results of a hearing test alone might as well be selling you snake oil.

Instead, high-quality treatment assesses not only the nature of your hearing loss, but also the hearing you need to do. Suppose two people have a similar hearing loss. As I implied before, the one who lives in an assisted-living facility has different hearing needs from the one who works in a fast-paced job requiring 35 hours a week of meetings. We all travel the same roads, but some of us need a minivan and others need a sports car, with many options in between. The same is true of hearing aids.

Even the size and shape of your ear canal plays a role. Remember that many providers rely on manufacturer-provided fitting software. The algorithm recommends the best and most comfortable fit based on your test results and average ear canal size. This method isn't anywhere close to adequate. The size and shape of *your* ear canal determines the performance of *your* hearing technology.

Imagine a pipe with water rushing through it. If you change the width of the pipe even slightly, you significantly increase or decrease the amount of water going through. Your ear canal is like a pipe that sound travels through. But unlike a pipe, your ear canal has curves and bends. If your hearing aid doesn't fit flush with your ear canal, sound leaks out. Your device won't perform as it should.

The Adjustment Period

If somebody's chief concern is making a sale, they are going to spend the period before the warranty expires making your device as comfortable as possible. Many companies only offer a 30-day return period for their products. That's far less time than you need. It's important to have enough time to determine if they're the right technology. You also need to allow your ears and brain to adapt to the new sounds. Aware of this issue, many manufacturers set up their programing software so the warranty period is spent making the devices more comfortable, not more effective. Thus, the manufacturer ensures a patient doesn't return the hearing aids during the warranty period.

You need a provider who insists on devoting time to determining the right treatment solution. They should educate you about your hearing loss and share their expertise. Hearing technology is a considerable investment. It should work as well as possible. Some practices do offer a longer warranty period than the manufacturer's guarantee. But that's a gamble not everyone can afford to take. Regardless of the warranty duration, you want somebody who's goal is adjusting the device is to make sure you hear as effectively as possible.

Validation Matters

Often I will ask patients with hearing technology if their hearing loss is well treated. Usually, the answer is "yes." I ask how they can tell. I usually get a puzzled look. In the same way a patient can't assess the nature of their hearing loss, they can't assess the quality of their treatment. Subjective first-person evaluations are simply not medically meaningful. It would be like telling your doctor, "I feel fine, so I don't think I have high blood pressure."

Accurate and personalized validation of hearing technology is the only way to gauge whether it's treating your hearing loss. At my practice, we use Arizona Hearing Real Ear Measurement to objectively assess hearing treatment.

"Accurate and personalized validation of hearing technology is the only way to gauge whether it's treating your hearing loss. At my practice, we use the Arizona Hearing Real Ear Measurement."

Real Ear Measurement measures the output of the hearing aid to ensure it provides the correct amplification for your hearing loss. A small microphone is placed in your ear canal along with the hearing aid (you don't even feel it) to measure how much volume the hearing aid provides. The key is that this step happens in *your* ear. Your fitting should be based on *your* ear canals, not a computer-generated guess.

You may recall that in Chapter 1, I mentioned a *Consumer Reports* study finding that two-thirds of hearing aids are not programmed correctly. That's because validation should be done in the context of the patient, rather than in a vacuum. A suit is tailored to a person, not a mannequin.

The Arizona Hearing Real Ear Measurement is compared to your personal audiogram to determine whether the hearing technology appropriately treats your hearing loss.

We treat medical problems with measurement. When you go to your primary care physician, your height, weight, pulse, blood pressure, temperature, and other data are collected. Your doctor doesn't simply look at you and say, "You look like your blood pressure is good." Measurement is essential on the pathway to quality.

Hearing Aids In A Drawer = Provider Failure

Unworn hearing technology isn't an effective treatment for hearing loss. No matter how good the model is in theory, it's useless in a nightstand drawer. Simply put, lack of use is a treatment failure. For example, if your primary care physician prescribes a blood pressure medicine and you don't take it, you're not receiving treatment. The same is true of hearing technology: If it's not worn, it can't work. And when patients don't wear hearing aids, it's because they don't see an improvement in their hearing lifestyle.

Make no mistake—this is a provider failure, not a patient failure.

Getting Away From Plug and Play

Now that we've seen what a great course of treatment looks like, let's return to that original analogy. You're presented with three hearing aid providers offering you the same range of devices.

The first is going to do some basic testing, recommend a model, make sure it does something—anything—for you, and call it a day.

The second is going to do a better job testing, ask you a little bit about yourself and your needs, choose the most suitable device they know of, fit it using good-but-not-great software, give you some time to tinker with the device, and then send you on your way.

> "Do not buy a hearing aid. Instead, *get your hearing loss treated*. Hearing care is not a plug and play. The quality of the provider has a direct impact on whether hearing devices will treat your hearing loss."

The third is going to test as comprehensively as possible (not using a prior hearing test performed elsewhere), take the time to talk about your listening lifestyle, educate you and your loved ones about your hearing loss, carefully select the most appropriate model (or models) for your needs, expertly fit the hearing aid to ensure maximum performance, validate the fit with Real Ear Measurement, and regularly make sure that standard of performance is maintained.

As with the masons, these services are priced accordingly. Many Arizona Hearing Center patients come to us with existing hearing technology, but they're frustrated with their hearing experience. Too often, their provider overpromised and under delivered. The patient was left wondering why there was no improvement.

It's no wonder so many people don't "like" their hearing aids. The devices we call hearing aids are commodities. Getting your hearing loss treated is a service. If you were offered a half-price surgery, you would seek care elsewhere. Services are judged based on quality. Who are you going to choose if you truly want your hearing loss treated well?

If you were to whittle my advice about treating hearing loss down to one nugget, it would have to be, "Go with the best." Do not buy a hearing aid. Instead, ***get your hearing loss treated.***

Hearing care is not a plug-and-play device that you can buy, unbox, and use. In fact, it's the furthest thing from it. The care and diligence you take in getting educated and selecting the best provider has a direct impact on whether your hearing devices will treat your hearing loss and improve your life.

CHAPTER 7

Instant Gratification Is Short Lived And Full Of Regret

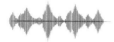

Alberto and Micky knew their 70-year-old father had become hard of hearing. He couldn't hear their mom at Sunday dinner, and he was becoming forgetful. The grandchildren were sad because grandpa couldn't hear them anymore during charades. No one in the family, including their father, wanted to put him in a nursing home. The two brothers agreed their dad needed help to improve his hearing and quality of life—but they disagreed about what help looked like.

Micky had seen the commercial. That same one where the senior angrily complains about the cost of hearing aids and how providers charge "anything they can get." Micky wanted to take their dad to Walmart to get the best price. He figured it was like buying a television or any other appliance. Micky wanted to help his dad as quickly as possible.

Alberto had a different idea. One of his friends struggled with hearing aids purchased at a big box retailer—they were very uncomfortable. Alberto wanted his dad to see an ear doctor for an evaluation, treatment recommendations, and a hearing-improvement plan.

But in the end, Micky convinced their dad to go to Walmart. Their dad walked out with new hearing aids that same day. After a month or two of struggling with them, what do you think happened? You guessed it—they ended up in the nightstand drawer. Dad was no closer to having his hearing loss treated.

Alberto knew his dad would be in much better shape if they had gotten his hearing loss **treated.** *Buying what Micky considered an appliance had been the wrong decision. This bad experience convinced their dad he was beyond help. It was almost impossible now for Alberto and Micky to get him to an experienced treatment provider. Alberto and Micky just wanted to help their dad live a better life. Everyone was frustrated, with no solution in sight.*

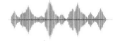

We live in an instant-gratification world. I can't fault people like Micky for their instinctive approach to a family member's hearing loss. He has a problem, he wants to fix it, and he wants to do it in the easiest, most cost-effective way possible. That's why the Walmart or big-box solution seems like the best option. You walk in, consult with someone, and walk out with hearing aids that promise to change your life. For most people, unfortunately, that promise remains unfulfilled.

With any task or goal, you can choose whether to focus on the result or the process. When you're results-oriented, you seek a certain outcome. If you achieve the result, you're successful. When you're process-oriented, you focus on the steps needed to achieve the goal. You ensure each step is done to the best of your ability, and you adapt as needed.

An obvious illustration of this is standardized testing. A results-oriented person might be tempted to cheat or otherwise manipulate the outcome. Provided they're not caught, they might get a great score, but won't have any more knowledge. The victory is hollow and only helps superficially. A process-oriented person studies the material and gains a familiarity with it. They may not get a perfect score, but they'll have an understanding that will last long after the test.

The same dichotomy applies to the way you approach hearing loss treatment. If you see treatment as a result—most often buying a hearing aid—you'll think treatment is over once that result occurs. But you need to view your treatment as a process, one that will continue for the remainder of your life. It's only with this perspective—starting from the evaluation process—that you'll get the most out of your treatment.

"I'm a cochlear implant candidate."

On a fairly regular basis, a patient will declare exactly what they need when they arrive at our practice. Before we've so much as looked inside their ears, they've determined the course of treatment and envisioned the outcome: A quick, minimally invasive surgery, and they'll be able to hear as good as new. In a later chapter, I'll discuss misconceptions about cochlear implants. I use this example to illustrate that being results-oriented, especially when you have a narrow definition of a successful result, sets you up for failure.

It would be unfair to say we don't have a result in mind when treating a patient's hearing loss. Our goal is just that: **We want you to hear as well as possible.** But we have to maintain an open mind about how to get there. "Science," says physicist Michio Kaku, "is about testable, reproducible evidence." And treating hearing loss is a science. We, as care providers, have to let the data from an evaluation lead us to a result. We can't use evaluation as a way to confirm the outcome we want. Anything less is doing the patient a disservice.

Results-oriented patients are a product of the prevailing discourse about hearing loss and its treatment. It's usually not their fault. If you have a hearing problem, our culture tells us, you get a hearing aid. That's it and that's all. If your hearing loss is really bad, a doctor may prescribe a cochlear implant. In either case, the focus ends up being about the outcome, not the issue at hand—treating hearing loss.

Test, Test, And Test Again

Treating hearing loss is not a perfect formula. We can't plug in a series of facts and figures based on a patient's condition and get a recipe for treatment. Treatment needs to be tested and adapted based on detailed evaluation of different facets of your auditory system. We have a wealth of technology to perform these evaluations, and the more testing we do, the better.

Hearing loss is not a condition you can shoehorn into a standard, pre-prescribed treatment. Again, treatment is a service. All good service providers tailor their approach to the person in front of them. You wouldn't go to a hair stylist who only specializes in one particular haircut. Why would you want hearing treatment from somebody who has decided beforehand they're going to sell you a hearing aid?

"At the diagnostic and information-gathering stages, the more data the better. That's why a successful outcome depends on finding the best and most thorough health care provider."

An effective route will only reveal itself through testing. What I'm advocating for is verification across the entire auditory system. Hearing is a complex physiological and neurological process. It should be standard practice to evaluate the ear canal, the eardrum, ear bones, the cochlea (hearing organ), the nerves, and the brain. It's different from saying, "Let's test your ears." At the diagnostic and information-gathering stages, the more data, the better. That's why a successful outcome depends on finding the best and most thorough hearing care provider.

Regular Reevaluation

At the diagnostic and information gathering stages, the more data, the better. That's why a successful outcome depends on finding the best and most thorough hearing care provider. Evaluation doesn't stop just because we've decided on a treatment. Consider a fitness regimen. You weigh yourself and perform basic tests before your first session. But it doesn't stop there. You repeat the weighing and testing regularly to monitor your progress. It's important to be process-oriented, but you can't trust the results of any process on blind faith.

Before wearing any hearing aid technology regularly, it needs to be programmed and validated by an expert. It's similar to a brace created for an athlete—it's rigorously tested and adjusted before the player ever steps on a field. Come game day, the device is as optimized as possible for its purpose. You can't simulate a game, of course, but it makes sense to get as close as possible.

After programming and validation, however, the evaluation process is far from over. Remember, your ears and brain have to adjust to hearing aids. The length of the adjustment period depends on the nature of the device. Regardless, you should undergo further evaluation after that period is complete. This is a critical crossroads where being process-oriented is essential. The convenience of you and your provider agreeing that the device needs no further tinkering comes at a price—better hearing. Ongoing evaluation is essential so you can report any issues and your provider can evaluate the effectiveness of your technology.

At every step, the intentions have to be the same: (1) Read detailed, comprehensive evaluation data objectively; (2) Assess the best possible course of action based on that individual data; and (3) Recover the appropriate amount of lost hearing for each patient's listening lifestyle. Making this goal a reality is a scientific process, which is to say it is one of continuous reevaluation.

CHAPTER 8

Understanding Your Hearing Test: Good Carpenters Measure Twice, Cut Once

If you've sought hearing loss treatment, you've probably seen test results in the form of an audiogram—a graph showing the softest sounds you can hear. This audiogram is only one small part of a comprehensive hearing evaluation. There are many different tests to evaluate your hearing, both with and without hearing technology. The craft of treating hearing loss requires a hearing professional to select and utilize the right battery of tests for each patient's specific situation.

> "The craft of treating hearing loss requires a hearing loss requires a hearing professional to select and utilize the right batter of tests for each patient's specific situation."

Our goal at Arizona Hearing Center is to enable our patients to hear as well as possible. This is rarely accomplished with just an audiogram.

I often meet patients with hearing aids who still have problems hearing and communicating. I ask, "Did your hearing aid provider confirm that your hearing has in fact improved?" The most common response is the patient's puzzled expression.

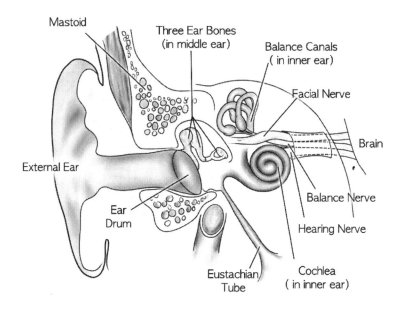

If all you have is a hammer, everything looks like a nail. If all you have is an audiogram, your patients will get subpar treatment. Let's take a look at the tools in the hearing professional's toolbox.

How Hearing Works

In order to better understand the testing, it's important to have a grasp of the basics of how hearing works.

Sound enters the ear canal and hits the eardrum. The eardrum vibrates and moves the three bones of hearing—the malleus, incus, and stapes. The stapes then vibrates the fluid in the cochlea, the organ of hearing. In the cochlea, structures called hair cells sense the waves in the fluid, convert them into nerve signals, and send the signals to the brain via the hearing nerve (called the cochlear nerve).

Audiogram: The EKG Of The Ear

If you grew up in the United States, you probably remember hearing screenings in your elementary school nurse's office. The specifics vary depending on state and era, but they probably went something like this: You sat down, and some very uncomfortable headphones were placed on your ears. The nurse asked you to raise the hand on the same side as the ear you heard a sound in. After a dozen or so beeps, you were done. It wasn't a particularly sophisticated screening test. Some of you probably even gamed it by listening for the nurse to flip the switch.

Thankfully, an audiogram isn't so easy to cheat. That's why it's become the customary test for audiological evaluation. It's an invaluable tool for analyzing a person's hearing. But it's not comprehensive—an audiogram needs to be interpreted by a professional and supplemented with additional testing.

The easiest comparison is the electrocardiogram, or EKG. The audiogram and the EKG are both screening tests that provide a detailed, relevant readout of your health. The EKG reflects your heart health; the audiogram, your hearing health. But if there's a problem, neither tool indicates a cause. An EKG can't tell you where a vessel is blocked, and an audiogram can't tell you what's causing your hearing loss. But they're both extremely effective measuring tools.

What does the audiogram measure, exactly? Your ability to hear a given range of frequencies.

You can think of frequency as pitch. Children, who tend to have high-pitched voices, speak at high frequencies. The deep rumble of an engine is a low pitch, or a low frequency.

During the audiogram test, you're presented with a range of frequencies from 125 Hz to 8,000 Hz (hertz, or cycles per second). The test administrator increases the volume step by step (measured in decibel, dB) until you indicate that you can hear it. The test is done separately for each ear, and the results are in the form of a graph. Usually, the right ear is represented by a red line with circles; the left ear, by a blue line with crosses.

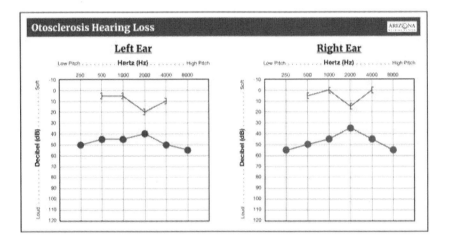

Reading Your Audiogram

Each circle or cross represents a tested frequency, and the lines connect each point. Across the top (*x*-axis) you see that the numbers (Hz, frequency or pitch) increase from left to right. But along the side (*y*-axis), you see that the numbers (dB, volume) increase from top to bottom. A large decibel number means the tester had to turn up the volume quite a bit before the sound was heard. Put another way, lots of volume means hearing loss. This is why the decibel numbers go from top to bottom, not bottom to top—visually, it suggests hearing loss.

A perfectly functioning ear will hear at a volume ranging from 0–25 dB. Mild hearing loss requires 25–40 dB; moderate hearing loss, 40–70 dB; severe hearing loss, 70–90 dB; and profound hearing loss, 90–120 dB. The horizontal location of the crosses and circles depends on how many tones are tested and the frequency of those tones. The horizontal position, however, will be the same for all patients who are tested using the same tones. The vertical positions vary by patients and for each ear.

The average audiogram almost always reflects a downward trend from left to right. That's because, as mentioned earlier when discussing golf legend Arnold Palmer, high frequencies are the first to go in almost all kinds of progressive hearing loss. If the general trend of your audiogram goes upward or fluctuates in the middle, it tells your audiologist you have a special case.

The audiogram actually tests two different hearing routes. One is the normal hearing mechanism, which tests how well you hear sound waves (air conduction). The second is from behind the ear directly to the hearing organ. This tests how well your bones conduct sound (yes, your bones conduct sound!). You process sounds both ways. If we can understand the viability of each, we can understand the precise nature of your hearing loss.

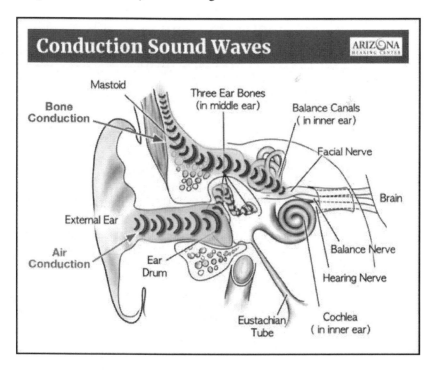

An audiogram will be performed both without and with hearing aids. In the latter case, this assesses the performance of specific models. In the course of treating your hearing loss, a lot of audiograms might be performed. But it's by no means a crystal ball that provides a perfect plan of action to treat your hearing loss.

Pitfalls Of An Audiogram

The biggest problem with an audiogram is it measures each ear independently. But your right ear does not work independently of your left ear, and vice versa. Unlike a Phil Spector recording or an early Beatles album, our world isn't in mono. Your ears are in constant conversation with each other as well as the outside world. There's a synergy there that isn't reflected in an audiogram. The same principle applies to hearing aids.

Does that mean, then, that you need two hearing aids? Yes. The second hearing aid will be an exponentially stronger investment than the first, simply because it will produce more than double the effect. The synergies work both ways, as it were.

Another shortcoming of an audiogram is it only measures how well you hear individual tones. But hearing is more than that. An audiogram can't tell whether you can understand speech. Hearing a 500-Hz tone is one thing; interpreting language at 500 Hz is another altogether.

Now, these shortcomings aren't problems in and of themselves. Very few medical tests are as definitive as a strep-throat swab. The problem arises when an audiogram is expected to do everything— such as when a hearing aid provider uses an audiogram and nothing else.

Patterns of Audiogram

The pattern of the audiogram indicates the cause of the hearing loss. A common pattern of hearing loss, second only to normal, is presbycusis, or age-related hearing loss. This pattern occurs in one of every three adults over the age of 65. The hearing is better in the low frequencies (for example, men's voices and thunder) and worse in the high frequencies (for example, children's voices and birds).

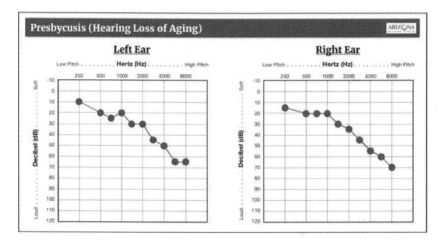

In patients with a severe hearing loss, the hearing is usually poor in all frequencies. This is an example of an audiogram for a patient with severe hearing loss. Remember, normal hearing takes place between 0 and 25 dB—this patient needed the volume to be turned up to between 70–90 dB.

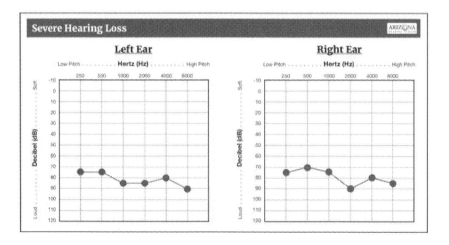

The chart indicates the levels of hearing loss and their descriptions.

Degrees of Hearing Loss
ARIZONA
HEARING CENTER

Type of Hearing Loss	In Decibels (dB)
Normal Hearing	-10 - 20
Mild Hearing Loss	20 - 40
Moderate Hearing Loss	40 - 60
Moderately Severe Hearing Loss	60 - 70
Severe Hearing Loss	70 - 90
Profound Hearing Loss	90 - 120

The prior two audiograms only show measurements for air conduction (sound waves). This is because the bone-conduction measurements were the same as those for the air conduction test. The following audiogram shows how it looks when there's a difference between the air-conduction and bone-conduction tests.

The bone-conduction values are normal, but the air-conduction values are between 40 dB and 55 dB. This tells me that a problem with the ear canal, eardrum, or ear bones (ossicles) is the cause of the hearing loss. The pattern of the bone loss can suggest the underlying cause of the bone-conduction hearing loss. In this example, the cause is secondary to otosclerosis. Otosclerosis is an abnormal bone growth that causes the stapes bones to become stiff.

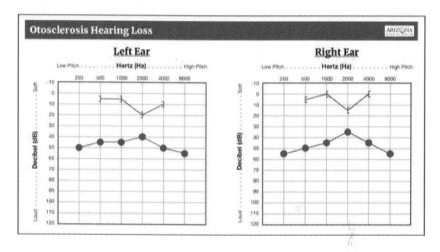

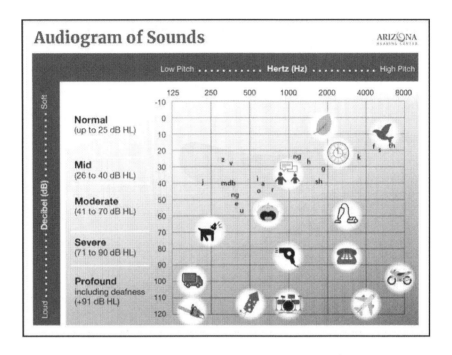

The above figure shows where various sounds fall on the audiogram. When a patient's measured hearing level is beneath a sound on the above diagram, they can't hear the sound. For example, someone with a severe hearing loss can only hear the sounds at the bottom of the diagram, such as a chainsaw, fireworks, drums, a jet, or a motorcycle.

Presbycusis creates a different problem. As the figure shows, vowels are low pitched and consonants are high pitched. Someone with presbycusis can hear vowels but has trouble hearing consonants. A common complaint is they can hear well, they just can't understand sometimes. They often accuse others of mumbling.

Supplementing An Audiogram

We use the audiogram as a tool to help diagnose exactly why you have the hearing loss you do. When multiple hearing-loss patients have the same underlying issue, it usually shows up as a pattern in each patient's audiogram. Learning and recognizing these patterns, thus, is helpful in determining the best course of action for you. But nobody can look at an audiogram alone and tell you, "Here is the exact hearing aid you need." It's a crucial piece of the puzzle, but don't be fooled into thinking it's the only one.

An audiogram has to be considered in light of other tests that provide more context and nuance about your condition. As a hearing care professional, I'd love to be able to rely on a single test to tell me exactly what's going on and what to do about it. But that's not the reality. Good care requires multiple tests that take all kinds of criteria into account.

Comprehension (Clarity) Testing

Hearing is more than simply registering the presence of a tone—you need to be able to understand a series of them. That's why, at Arizona Hearing Center, we use an auditory comprehension test to clarify the results of your audiogram. During this exam, you hear words and then try to repeat them back to us. This helps determine whether you're experiencing cognitive impairment because of your hearing loss. It also tests your ability to hear a series of different frequencies in succession. After all, you never hear isolated tones in the real world.

Furthermore, clarity and volume are two distinct hearing phenomena—you can't have clarity without volume, but volume doesn't guarantee clarity. In other words, sometimes we can get the volume where it needs to be for you, but you can't understand the sounds any better. Understanding nuances like these in individual hearing loss is vital to creating a course of treatment.

Arizona Hearing Real Ear Measurement

As mentioned earlier, Real Ear Measurement measures the output of the hearing aid to validate that it provides the correct amplification for your hearing loss. A small microphone is placed in your ear canal along with the hearing aid (you don't even feel it) to measure how much volume the hearing aid provides. The key is that this step happens in *your* ear. Your fitting should be based on *your* ear canals, not a computer-generated guess. The Arizona Real Ear Measurement is compared to your audiogram to determine whether the hearing technology appropriately treats your hearing loss.

Functional Testing

One way an audiogram can be misleading is that it happens outside of real-world conditions. Obviously, the testing booth is important to provide a clear baseline of your hearing free of interference.

"Many new patients tell me hearing devices they got elsewhere worked great at the hearing treatment center but poorly at home. That's because the devices weren't programmed for real-world conditions."

However, you'll never use your hearing technology in a hearing-testing booth in your day-to-day life. It's crucial to simulate conditions similar to those in which you'll be using your devices.

Let's go back to the EKG comparison. A patient tells their doctor, "I have chest pain when I go up the stairs." The doctor will start by running an EKG—but that test is done in resting conditions. An EKG may not indicate a problem, even if it's there. Often, the cardiologist also performs a stress test to assess the patient's heart during exercise.

The same is true of your hearing. The audiogram tells us one thing, functional testing tells us another. Many new patients tell me the hearing devices they got elsewhere worked great at the hearing treatment center but poorly at home. That's because the provider didn't do functional testing – the devices weren't programmed for real-world conditions. Ideally, this testing is done using both hearing aids simultaneously as well as in background noise.

Cognitive Testing

Hearing is the detection of sound. Communication is the imparting or exchanging of information. As described earlier, the brain is an essential component of communication, but technology can only deliver the information to the brain. In some patients, communication is still a problem. In these circumstances, we perform cognitive screening and, if warranted, refer the patient for further evaluation and treatment. Often, effectively treating a patient's hearing is one of the first steps in treating their cognitive problems.

We use other tests as well, depending on the patient, but the goal is always to get the most detailed picture possible from both a diagnostic and treatment perspective. Testing needs to determine both how a patient's hearing loss is affecting them and how the treatment technology is performing.

CHAPTER 9

One Size Does Not Fit All: Especially When It Comes To Your Hearing Health

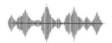

I have a son and two daughters, so I've long been aware of certain expenses looming. Piano and dance lessons, athletics, summer camp, and tuition were all in my future. When my eldest, Matthew, was 11, we found out he needed braces. The memories came rushing back—the metal, the rubber bands, the headgear, and, of course, the occasional snide "metal mouth" comment. I felt a little bad for the kid.

But the technology had advanced a lot. I was assured Matthew would only have to wear braces for a year, which was, indeed, how it turned out. He ended up having a much easier time than I did. He was fitted with braces, dutifully followed instructions, switched to retainers after six months, and boom—he now has a camera-ready smile that even George Clooney would envy.

"Wow," I thought. "That experience wasn't so bad."

Until it was my daughter Meredith's turn. Her case was a little more complicated. Because she had a narrow palate, she had to be fit with a palate widener. We had to crank it every day for a few months before she could receive her braces—which she had to wear for two years. What I didn't know at the time was that Meredith, out of frustration about the time frame, had taken matters into her own hands. She had doubled up on the rubber bands that went with her braces, so she managed to cut her time down by six months! Meredith always has been an over-achiever...

My youngest daughter, Marinna, is still waiting for her braces, but her case is even more complicated. Her adult teeth are delayed, and it looks like she might need some baby teeth pulled. She will probably need a palate widener, her braces will need to stay on longer because of her overbite, and she might need to wear headgear at night.

I was naïve to think orthodontia would be standard for all of them. Like most things having to do with my children, one size does not fit all—even with something that seems straightforward, like braces. If you want to get it right, you have to make sure you're using the correct tools for each person's case.

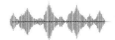

Alternative Technology for Particular Hearing Loss Cases

Like my children's braces, hearing health is not a one-size-fits-all proposition. There are thousands of traditional hearing aid models available. Each addresses slightly different hearing issues. They work by using a speaker to push sound waves through your ear canal to your eardrum. Known as air conduction, this method can treat most people's hearing loss.

But air-conduction hearing aids can't meet the needs of some people with hearing loss. Many of these patients throw up their hands and go without. Others settle for something that doesn't help and ends up unused in the nightstand drawer. The good news is there are other potential solutions.

These alternatives are not better or worse than air-conduction hearing aids. Discussing alternatives with your provider is part of educating yourself — you're not inviting an upsell. Each patient has unique hearing health care needs. For some, the best solution is a device that uses a different kind of technology.

The Limits of Traditional Hearing Aids

We live in a world where technology squeezes more power into smaller spaces. The same processing power we have in our smartphones would have required warehouses of huge computers decades ago. We can minimize the space needed for our tech, but we can't eliminate it. And one area where spatial confines are important is hearing aid design.

Air-conduction hearing aids are, essentially, a microphone, a processor, and a speaker. The microphone and speaker must be placed in the hearing aid in a certain way. But that placement limits their volume and range of frequency. This, in a nutshell, is the challenge of hearing aid design.

Volume

Remember the daily announcements over your school's PA system? When you heard feedback, that was because the microphone got too close to one of the speakers. In the same way, designers of air-conduction hearing aids have to keep the microphone and speaker far enough apart to avoid feedback — but they have to do it in a tiny hearing aid. This is why the microphone on so many air-conduction hearing aids is placed behind the ear. In small, discreet devices that sit entirely in the ear canal, the microphone has to be placed very close to the speaker. In order to fight the resulting feedback, the hearing aid's processor has to sacrifice volume performance. But loss of functional hearing is too big a price to pay for aesthetic benefit.

Frequency Range

Frequency range also limits air-conduction hearing aids, which take in sounds via the microphone, process them, and reproduce them with the speaker. The designers of these devices want to capture as wide a range of sounds as possible, but they also want to reproduce those sounds clearly and faithfully.

And that's why a compromise is necessary. As the range of frequencies being input gets wider, clearly reproducing all those sounds in the ear canal gets more difficult. It's a bit like a flashlight or a car headlight — the wider the beam, the less bright and focused the light is.

So, air-conduction hearing aid designers have to find that sweet spot between ample input and clear output. In this case, on average, it's a frequency range of 500 Hz to 5,000–6,000 Hz. Normal human speech falls within this range. And that's what most people need a hearing aid to do — communicate.

There are always outliers for whom air-conduction hearing aids aren't a viable solution. In these exceptional situations, other classes of technology can address their hearing problem.

Earlens: A Different Kind of Hearing Aid

In the past three decades, Silicon Valley has been an innovator and disruptor. It has put an end to typewriters, video stores, and printed maps, to name a few. So why not traditional hearing aids as well?

Because hearing aid technology is an engineering problem without an easy solution. The major industry players have a wealth of experience and R&D resources, but hearing aids are still alive and well. There is hope, though. Some companies are radically challenging the notion of what a hearing aid can be. One of those companies is the tech company Earlens.

Earlens

Founded in 2005 by Dr. Rodney Perkins, Earlens produces a different kind of hearing aid. It transmits sound, but not in the standard way. Instead of using air conduction, the Earlens uses electromagnetic conduction. This process captures a wider range of frequencies, providing a more faithful, natural, less compromised hearing experience. In practice, this allows you to hear sounds you wouldn't hear with a traditional hearing aid. As one Earlens user commented, "I can now hear the violins clearly when I go to the symphony, while I could hardly hear them at all before."

Many who wear air-conduction hearing aids experience voices as electronic or robotic. The new design of the Earlens provides more natural-sounding, authentic voices. This increases the likelihood that patients will actually use the hearing aids.

How Earlens Works

A custom-built, thin silicone lens with a magnet is fitted against — not attached to — your eardrum. The Earlens microphone picks up sound, processes it, and sends a current down a thin rod in your ear canal. At the end of the rod is a coil that converts the current into a magnetic field. The magnet in the silicon lens picks up the vibrations of the magnetic field and transfers those vibrations to your eardrum.

As you can see, this is very different from air conduction, in which sound waves travel through the air toward your eardrum to make it vibrate.

A Promising Alternative

The distance between the microphone and the sound production is much greater in an Earlens hearing aid, so it can provide more volume without creating feedback. At Arizona Hearing Center, we see many patients who can't get the volume they need with air-conduction hearing aids — for them, the Earlens is an excellent option.

Many patients want to test-drive the Earlens before they commit to a custom-made product. Fortunately, at Arizona Hearing Center, we are able to provide that comparison so patients can hear for themselves how Earlens is an improvement over their current hearing aids.

Let's move from the relative newcomer Earlens to another form of hearing technology, one with a longer history that meets a different need entirely.

Cochlear Implants and a Different Way of "Hearing"

The Hair Cell

As mentioned before, your inner ear has a structure called a cochlea. Hair cells in your cochlea receive sound, translate it into nerve impulses, and send the impulses to your brain.

Some people have hair cells that don't work. This could be from a birth defect, trauma, or other reasons. In these situations, the cochlea can't send sound information to the brain. You can use hearing aids or Earlens to send sound to your cochlea, but the sound will stop there—the damaged hair cells can't relay the message. What if we could somehow bypass the hair cells entirely?

The Cochlear Implant

A cochlear implant skips the hair cells. It goes to the next step in the hearing process—the auditory nerve—and uses electrical signals to stimulate it directly. Even if your hearing structures don't function at all, a cochlear implant could be a viable option.

The device has both external and internal components. The external component is normally worn behind your ear. The internal component is the actual implant, which is surgically placed under your scalp under general anesthesia. The surgery is routine and minimally invasive. It is not, however, a cure-all by itself. To ensure success, a cochlear-implant patient must be diligent, and they must be well-informed by their health care provider.

The Challenges of Wearing a Cochlear Implant

A cochlear implant might seem like an easy win. "You mean my hearing, no matter how broken, can be corrected? You're telling me we can stimulate the auditory nerve directly, so I don't need traditional hearing aids? Sign me up!" If it were that simple, everyone with hearing loss would choose cochlear implants. It's a remarkable piece of technology, but it doesn't work miracles in all cases. The cochlear implant team must educate the candidate on the challenges they'll face.

With a cochlear implant, you have to learn to hear in an entirely new way. You're going from acoustical hearing, which you've done your entire life, to electrical hearing—an entirely new cognitive process. If you hope to wake up with the volume just right and the clarity tuned to perfection, you're in for a rude awakening.

Learning this new process is difficult. People new to cochlear implants experience disorientation and difficulty comprehending speech. These are perfectly normal results, but if you don't know about them beforehand, it can be extremely discouraging. Expecting a cochlear implant to do something it cannot do leads to frustration and disillusionment.

You need to go into the process with complete awareness of the challenges you'll face. Much like physical therapy, cochlear implant patients have to "work out" with their new hearing system. But also like physical therapy, they have the help and support of a health care team.

Though I have performed thousands of cochlear implant surgeries, the best people to tell you what to expect are the patients themselves. One person who can provide a first-hand account is Robert Miller, a cochlear implant patient I treated. Here is how Robert describes the experience:

> *"I could tell my wife was talking to me or people were talking to me, but I couldn't define the whole. You're straining all the time to try to hear and you know it's a nuisance to say "What?" all the time. Each day since the activation [of my cochlear implant], my hearing has gotten better."*
> *– Robert Miller, Arizona Healing Center patient*

I tell my patients to see the cochlear implant process as similar to the wedding process. The day you decide to move forward as a candidate, you're engaged to that implant. Before the wedding day, you should get to know that implant as best you can. And like a marriage, the success of your relationship doesn't depend on what happens on your wedding day. Success comes from the work you put in each day to ensure your relationship lasts. Your cochlear implant can be a miracle for you, as long as you go about the process the right way.

Determining Cochlear Implant Candidacy

Medicare doesn't cover traditional hearing aids, but it does cover cochlear implants. Commodity-minded patients often approach qualifying for cochlear implants in the same way they approach getting into college. Thankfully, there's no way to beef up your extracurricular activities to make the cut for a cochlear implant. The only way you'll qualify is through extensive testing.

Even when a cochlear implant candidate is referred to us, we still put them through our battery of evaluations. The only result I care about is making sure a patient has the best hearing possible. I'm only going to clear a person for a cochlear implant if I believe it is the best treatment method for their needs.

We also see patients who become cochlear implant candidates over time. "If I'm going to be a candidate eventually," you may wonder, "why don't I just wait it out?" There are a number of reasons. First, there's no way to predict whether you'll become an implant candidate. Second, treating your hearing loss early may delay or eliminate the need for an implant. Third, treating hearing loss now can help prevent later health complications that often lead to nursing home care, such as Alzheimer's and dementia. Finally, you deserve to hear better today, not at some yet-to-arrive date.

What All Technology Has in Common

It's easy to see only the differences between traditional hearing aids, the Earlens, and cochlear implants. As a patient, you want to know why you might opt for one over the other. But there are aspects that are the same across the board. Most importantly, each is only a tool — without education from your care provider and buy-in from you, they won't work as well as they should. None of the technology that we use to treat hearing loss is automatic. Success will depend largely on you.

CHAPTER 10

Your Frequently Asked Questions Answered

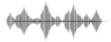

Over the course of my years in practice, I've heard patients bring up the same concerns over and over. It's a shame even the most basic aspects of hearing care aren't common knowledge. This chapter—indeed this entire book—is an attempt to close that education gap. This quick-reference guide is for those seeking answers to their questions about hearing loss and treatment. I hope you'll refer to it both when you have questions about hearing loss and when your loved ones do. If you have a question that is not answered, please email your questions or comments to: drsyms@ drmarksyms.com.

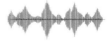

What brand and model of hearing aid should I buy?

First and foremost, making a purchase is not the same thing as treating hearing loss. Unlike buying a TV or a frying pan, your hearing loss isn't going to be resolved through a simple transaction. Hearing technology requires proper programming and patient education to work optimally.

There are thousands of models of hearing aids on the market, with new devices being released all the time. None of these is the best-in-class option for all patients. The question is exponentially more complex than asking, "What kind of car should I buy?" It simply can't be answered in any other way than on an individual basis.

To put it in stark terms, don't think of your treatment as "buying a hearing aid." You should follow the treatment plan recommended by a dedicated expert who has thoroughly assessed your hearing loss.

Why doesn't Medicare pay for hearing aids?

Medicare was first passed into law in 1965. In those days, hearing aids were sold by door-to-door salesmen—the same folks who peddled globes and encyclopedias. The government, for obvious reasons, wasn't going to line the pockets of people clearly outside the medical community.

The way that we think of and treat hearing loss has evolved significantly since then, but one residual effect is that for the vast majority of Americans, hearing loss treatment isn't covered by Medicare.

Do I need one hearing aid or two?

If you have hearing loss in both ears, you'll have a markedly better experience with two hearing aids. Furthermore, the degree to which you'll do better is even greater than you might expect. Two ears are better than one, and two hearing aids are better than one. The effect, however, isn't additive, but rather synergistic—in this case, one plus one doesn't equal two, it equals something more like four.

How should I clean my ears?

You shouldn't. Under no circumstance should you ever stick anything in your ears. If you look on a box of cotton swabs, you'll notice it says nothing about using them to clean your ears.

Earwax is natural, and ears are self-cleaning. Simply by chewing, your jaw muscles move excess earwax outside of your ear canal. You can use soap to wipe away any wax that forms outside of the ear canal, but there's no reason to clean the inside of it.

One reason people are tempted to clean their ears is a wet sensation that occurs after showering. To get rid of this feeling, you can simply hold a blow dryer at arm's length and dry out your ear canals.

Why can't I tell I have a hearing loss?

You don't know what you can't hear. Your brain is sophisticated and helps you compensate for the early stages of hearing loss. In fact, your early-stage hearing loss might be empirical—meaning I can detect it with a test—but you could probably still communicate nearly as effectively as somebody with normal hearing. However, over time, your progressive hearing loss will make it difficult to communicate.

Similarly, in the early stages, your hearing loss might feel situational. I say "feel" because it's present all the time. It only affects your ability to communicate in certain situations. Usually, the first places you'll notice communication problems will be public spaces, such as restaurants, and when your attention is divided, such as driving.

How should I ask other people to speak to me if I have a hearing loss?

I would recommend not telling people, especially strangers, that you have a hearing loss. Why? Their natural reaction will be to speak louder, which won't help you understand them. Instead, say you didn't understand what they just said.

For whatever reason, when you frame your response this way, they're more likely to rephrase their question. This gives you more context as well as a second chance to understand.

Compare these two interactions:
Spouse 1: Honey, what do you want for dinner?
Spouse 2: What? I didn't hear you.
Spouse 1: I said HONEY, WHAT DO YOU WANT FOR DINNER?

Or

Spouse 1: Honey, what do you want for dinner?
Spouse 2: Sorry, I didn't understand that.
Spouse 1: What would you like to eat?

How do I get a loved one to treat their hearing loss?

Broaching the topic of treatment with a loved begins by being honest. Tell them how their hearing loss affects you. Too many people present it as an entirely selfless request. They'll ask, "Don't you want to do it for yourself?" The problem here is it gives the person with hearing loss a way out—they might not, in fact, want to do it for themselves.

When somebody doesn't treat their hearing loss, it most strongly affects the people closest to them. You need to make that clear to your loved one with hearing loss. To be blunt, having to support somebody who refuses to treat their hearing loss is a burden. You can pretend otherwise, but it's not going to get you anywhere.

If honest dialogue won't get the job done, get your own hearing tested and bring your loved one along. I've found that this strategy works especially well with spouses. Simply getting them in an office removes a major barrier to treatment. It also demystifies the process, allowing them to see that audiological testing is a normal medical procedure like any other.

Can you cure tinnitus?

Tinnitus, the clinical term for hearing a sound that's not present, can't be cured. But that's no reason to avoid treatment—like diabetes, we can manage it. We can lessen the negative impact on your life. In fact, many patients experience a significant degree of relief through treatment. We can't cure some of the most common diseases in America. We shouldn't expect any different for tinnitus, but there is relief through management.

When is the best time to treat my hearing loss?

Yesterday! You should reconnect with the world as soon as possible. You treat age-related vision problems with reading glasses because it helps YOU see better. But the reason you treat your hearing loss is so THEY, your loved ones and friends, can connect with you better.

How is total hearing loss in one ear treated?

Four problems arise when hearing is completely lost in one ear. The most obvious is you can't hear in one ear. But you also can't hear as well in background noise, you have a much harder time determining where a sound is coming from, and you turn your head so you can hear the speaker better with your hearing ear. This means you're no longer looking straight into the speaker's eyes.

The strategy for treating this hearing loss is to capture the sound on the non-hearing side and transmit it to the hearing ear. If done wirelessly, this is called a CROS hearing aid system. If the sound is transmitted via the person's skull (through bone conduction), a surgically implanted device called a BAHA is used. The appropriate device is selected based on an assessment of the status of the hearing ear.

Can I really expect to be more socially engaged after treating my hearing loss?

Yes, yes, yes! If you weren't the life of the party before hearing loss, however you still likely won't be after hearing loss treatment. Hearing loss slowly leads to social withdrawal, but treating your hearing loss will enable you to socialize more and more easily. But don't just take it from me. Hear what one of our Arizona Hearing Center patients has to say:

> "It's a shame I waited so long to investigate [my hearing loss options]. If only I had treated it years back. I was a substitute teacher at the elementary school and...[hearing loss] always held me back from improving myself. You shut yourself out even to your friends and your family. You just don't feel like you're a part of anything. I thought I'd have to die like this but then we found Arizona Hearing Center and it's been remarkable to be able to hear like I do! I can hear someone in the next room. I couldn't before. Now I'm a part of everything!"
>
> ~Bonnie Grimm, patient of Dr. Mark J. Syms, MD
> and Arizona Hearing Center

Who are some famous people who have treated their hearing loss?

There are many famous people who have suffered from hearing loss, including Ronald Reagan, George Bush, Bill Clinton, Jodie Foster, Halle Berry, Pete Townshend, Marlee Matlin, Holly Hunter, Adam Savage, John Howard, Huey Lewis, Roger Daltrey, Eric Clapton, Whoopi Goldberg, Luis Miguel, Lou Ferrigno, Rob Lowe, Stephen Colbert, Rush Limbaugh, Jane Lynch, Robert Redford, Rikki Poynter, Millicent Simmonds, Thomas Edison, Will.i.am, Grimes, William Shatner, Derrick Coleman, Russell Harvard, Neil Young, Moby, Kiefer Sutherland, Lars Ulric, and Ludwig van Beethoven, to name a few.

Hearing loss does not have to stand in the way of you leading a highly successful life. You no longer have to suffer in silence. With a comprehensive hearing loss treatment plan from an expert hearing healthcare provider, you can maintain a vibrant and independent lifestyle filled with family, friends and all the activities you love

BIOGRAPHY

Dr. Mark Syms is a national leader in hearing technology and one of the first physicians in the country to be board certified in neurotology. He specializes in otology/neurotology and leads Arizona Hearing Center, an organization dedicated to treating hearing loss. He describes himself as the "E" of "ENT."

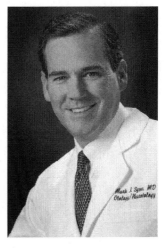

With more than two decades of experience treating ear problems, he helps tens of thousands of people improve their quality of life with better hearing. Dr. Syms is "The Hearing Loss Physician."

Dr. Syms graduated with honors from Boston College with degrees in biology and philosophy. He earned his medical degree from Jefferson Medical College and completed his ENT residency training at Tripler Regional Medical Center in Honolulu, HI, where he treated and saved the lives of many of our heroic veterans. He did his fellowship training at the House Ear Clinic in Los Angeles, one of the world's premier surgery organizations. Dr. Syms lectures frequently on neurotology locally, nationally, and internationally, is an extensively published author, and is a leader and member of numerous professional organizations.

Dr. Syms was born and raised in Philadelphia. He lives in Arizona with his wife, Maria, and their three children, Matthew, Meredith, and Marinna. In his free time, he enjoys movies, hiking, skiing, and spending time with his family and their dog, Maizie.

ACKNOWLEDGEMENT

Maria M. Syms, Matthew J. Syms, Meredith S. Syms, Marinna P. Syms, Charles A. Syms, Jr., MD, Kathryn Lynch Syms, Pasquale Mazzeo, Joyce Mazzeo, Charles A. Syms, III, MD, John P. Syms, Robert S. Syms, David W. Syms, Kathie S. McCauley, Bernise Lynch, Paul Mazzeo, MD, Francis Gradel, William Rumpf, Michael J. Bransfield, Brian Haley, Kevin Dalmasse, FSC, The La Salle Forum, Michael O'Toole, Arthur Burke, Joseph Leibrandt, Jeffrey Clarke, Carl Waldspurger, PhD, Mark Oberholzer, Greg Olbrich, Daniel Pickard, William Regli, PhD, Timothy Fighera, William Sullivan, SJ, Eleanor O'Brien, Ph.D., Ronald Tacelli, SJ, Joseph Healy, Kristin Lindemann, Brian Tierney, Thomas Kenny, Joseph Gonella, MD, Murray Cohen, MD, Frank Rossato, MD, Louis D. Lowry, MD, William M. Keane, Chadran Kalyanam, MD, Jay Jawad, MD, David Manuel, MD, Kimberly Jones, MD, Netra Thakur, MD, Hermann Moreno, MD, Michael Holtel, MD, Lawrence Burgess, MD, Donald Yim, MD, Mark Sheridan, MD, Florence Uyehara, Mitchell Ramsey, MD, Steven Suk, MD, Paulus Tsai, MD, Eugene Stec, MD, Jeffrey Hull, MD, Rick Visor, MD, Richard Bailey, MD, Pauline Mashima, James Sheehy, MD, Derald Brackmann, MD, Jennifer Dereberry, MD, William Luxford, MD, John House, MD, Howard House, MD, William House, MD, Antonio Dela Cruz, MD, Ralph Nelson, MD, William Slattery, MD, Fred Linthicum, MD, Marlan Hansen, MD, Elizabeth Toh, MD, Raoul Nucci, MD, Bradley Kesser, MD, Stephanie Moody Antonio, MD, Marlan Hansan, MD, William Hitselberger, MD, Clough Shelton, MD, Prescious Javiar, Rosie Morales, Douglas Backous, MD, Fred Telischi, MD, Bruce Gantz, MD, Craig Buchman,

MD, Richard Cole, MD, Hilary Brody, MD, Peter Weber, MD, Lawrence Lustig, MD, Anil Lalwani, MD, Robert Jackler, MD, Nikolas Blevins, MD, Eben Rosenthal, MD, Paul Howard, MD, Harold Pillsbury, MD, Randall Ow, MD, Seth Schwartz, MD, Brian McKinnon, MD, Patrick Antonelli, MD, Jose Fayad, MD, Sujana Chandrasekhar, MD, David Haynes, MD, Joseph Sniezek, MD, Michael Seidman, MD, Dennis Bojrad, MD, Neil Sperling, MD, Neil Giddings, MD, Stephen Cass, MD, Fred Telischi, MD, Peter Roland, MD, Terry Fife, MD, Guido Hattendorf, Randall Porter, MD, Michael Lawton, MD, Robert Spetzler, MD, Francisco Ponce, MD, Peter Nakaji, MD, Michael J.A. Robb, MD, Keith Bahlmann, Derrick Murphy, Richard Houseworth, Dean Howard, Timothy Louis, Christine Jones, John Asher, Marcia Asher, Robb Tyler, Jeff LeMaster, Greg Thielen, Jason Rose, Kevin Donlin, Emily Lawson, David Weinstock, PhD, Jean Moog, Bruce Rosenfield, Pam MacMillan, Rick MacMillan, Mal Jozoff, Jane Jozoff, Jini Simpson, Bob Hobbs, Karen Hobbs, Bob Parsons, Fife Symington, Marci Symington, Governor Fife Symington, Benjamin Hill, Alejandra Sota, Ross Meglathery, Anne MacDonald, Anders Graugaard, Adam LaReau, Simon Bone, Clay Coffeen, Besty Coffeen, Lou Vergne, Max Fose, Colin Shipley, Mark Goldman, Lisa Helt, Jamie Helt, Barbara Julian, Tom Palmer, Julie Palmer, Anette Reichman, Clara Walker, Lou Werner, Lea Werner, Jeff Ireland, Brandon Dawson, Mason Walker, Mike Halloran, J. Connon Samuel, Greg Damico, Chadwick Schneider, Laura Ramirez, Cynthia Sanchez, YanYan Bach, Jackie Crowder, Aric Burke, Vaughn Ward, Eric Boon, Iris Ross, Chuck Brown, Ryan Aldridge, Jennifer Ratigan, AuD, Kelly Hernandez, AuD, Shanna Mortensen, AuD, Cathy Kurth, AuD, Julie Darland, AuD, Judy Wong, AuD, Chris Writer, AuD, Christine Menapace, Teresa Adkins, Anthony Manna, Chris Smith, Chris Roberts, Patricia Trautwein, AuD, Anthony Arnold, Lalita Doughman, AuD, Jeffrey Greiner, Donna Sorkin, Drew Dundas,

PhD, William Facteau, Phil Lyons, Amir Abolfathi, Peter Hadrovic, Farris Walling, AuD, Victoria Roberts, Jerry Schloffman, David Morris, Rodney Perkins, MD, Susan Van Horne, John Vogrin, Julie Higginson, Paula Dyhrkopp, AuD, John White, Cellina Perez, Adriana Ponce, Gladis Ramos, Christina Pepa, Ceciley Villegas, Della Tao, Shelly Baltodano, AuD, Kory Castro, Taylor Kuminkoski, AuD, Rosie Villegas, Linda Vanderbeek, PA, Jay Heiler, Laryn Callaway, Christian Block, Gianna Bickson, Michael Bickson, Marinna Crosetti, Cindy Crosetti, Tina Richter, Jerry Cobb, Katie Cobb, Joseph DiGrigoli.

All have contributed along the way to help me formulate the content of this book and help me to be the best physician possible.

Made in the USA
Columbia, SC
28 October 2020